Side Effects

Other books by Jimmie Ashcraft, M.D.

Reflections of a Country Doctor

The Next Prescription

Side Effects

Another Dose of Stories
by a Country Doctor

Jimmie Ashcraft, M.D.

second printing revised edition 2020

Country Doctor Books
2437 Eastridge Drive
Billings, MT 59102

ISBN: 978-1-7345193-6-5

This book is printed on acid free paper.

Cover design by David Ashcraft

In Memory of

Georgia Fischer, R.N.

1953 - 2012

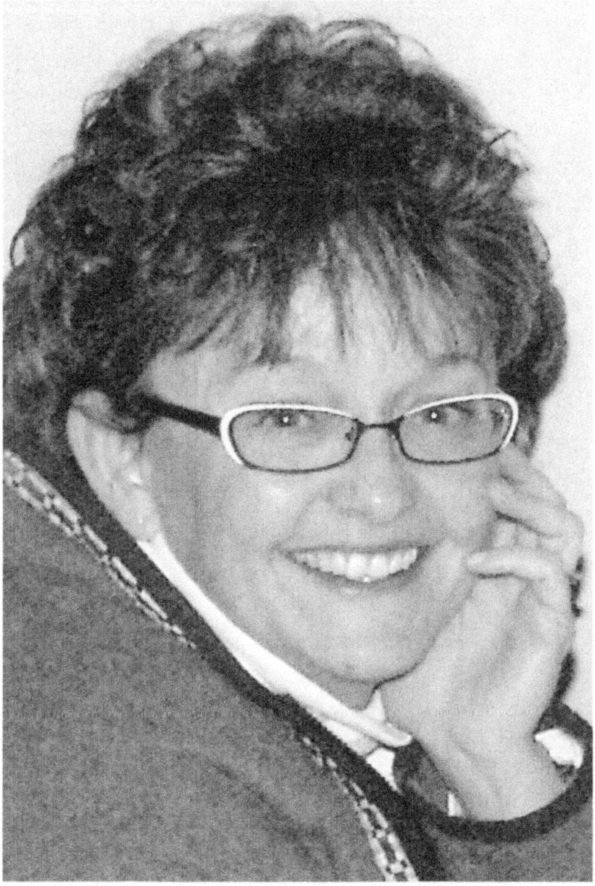

Georgia Fischer, R.N. was my office nurse for many years after I started private practice in Sidney, Montana. She was involved with many of my stories. Georgia crafted the rock doctor figurine shown on the book's cover which started my collection. Unfortunately, Georgia was a victim of a medical side effect and died too young. We all will miss her.

To

my wife Kay

our children

and

our grandchildren

Contents

Acknowledgements

Remembering events and retelling them in detail has always been easy for me. However, I found that the process of putting my verbal stories into a written language other than medical speak that others can understand is quite a challenge. For the possibility of even attempting this effort, I owe many.

The people who allowed me the privilege of caring for them over the many years deserve my utmost gratitude. Obviously, without them, I would not have as many memories to share or stories to tell.

I must salute my mentors, colleagues, dedicated office staff, and friends through the years, each of whom, in their own way, left a piece of themselves with me.

One group of individuals, Richard and Mary Woods, Diane Cross, and Jeff Nesset, were willing to read my text and offer editing suggestions along with constructive criticisms on how to convert medical speak into something readable have my utmost gratitude.

My daughter Becky made the original computer database of my patients years ago. That database along with my charts and memory provided the backbone for these stories.

Hugs and kisses are due to my children, Jennifer, Becky, and David, who encouraged me to write more of my stories and offered excellent suggestions for the cover design.

Finally, one person has been at my side through all the parts in this book: my wife Kay. She knows most of the stories and read, edited, and provided invaluable suggestions for the manuscript multiple times. I could not have accomplished this endeavor without her.

Author's Note

The stories in this book are true. I have done my best to portray the episodes as accurately as my memory and records would allow. To protect people's confidentiality, I have changed the names of individuals, my patients, their families, and my colleagues. I have changed details that might identify certain people or places.

“Laughter is a tranquilizer with no side effects”

Arnold H. Glasow
American businessman, humorist

Prologue

I have had the good fortune of being a part of medicine in one way or another for over four decades. During that time, I have seen advances in science that even to my most progressive thinking medical school mentors would seem unfathomable. All too often I appreciated how quickly old ideas and methods were discarded by colleagues when newer ones developed, only to find out later than the old way was often the better way, or the older drug, although out of favor for a time, was a better treatment.

Sir William Osler (1849-1919), a Canadian physician considered by many to be the father of modern medicine and one of the four original founders of the Johns Hopkins Hospital and Medical School, astutely noted: "A look at the past will show that the philosophies of one age become the absurdities of the next, and the foolishness of yesterday becomes the wisdom of tomorrow."

Many common maladies today's physician confronts are the same illnesses that physicians have tried to cure since ancient times. The common cold, for example, is a viral infection that is just as incurable today as it was in the time of Hippocrates (c460 B.C. - c370 B.C.). To treat the cold, physicians today recommend rest, fluids, fresh air, and frequent hand washing.

Comparing our modern treatment for the common cold with that recommended by Dr. John Tennent, a colonial Virginia practitioner (c1700-1765), in his book, Every Man His Own Doctor: OR, The Poor Planter's Physician, which was printed in 1734 by Benjamin Franklin, we find little difference.[1]

"I shall begin with a COUGH, which is the foundation of many distempers, and therefore should be taken care of soon as possible. It may be cured in the beginning with riding moderately on horseback every day, and only taking a little Ground Ivy Tea sweetened with Syrup of Horehound, at night when you go to bed. In the mean while, you must use a spare and cooling diet, without either flesh or strong drink. Nor should you stove yourself up in a warm room, but breathe as much as possible in the open air. And to prevent mischief, don't make yourself tender, but wash every day in cold water, and very often your feet."

Physicians too often overlook the medical knowledge and observations from antiquity. The origins of many treatments and medicines we use today can be found in centuries past. Opium, for example, was used around 4000 B.C. for the relief of pain, anxiety, diarrhea, and a multitude of other ailments. [2] Around 1900 Sir William Osler called opium, "God's Own Medicine." This plant is the basis for today's arsenal of narcotic analgesics. One of its earliest products, tincture of opium or laudanum, still is used occasionally today.

Other old remedies that remain in use today, either in herbal preparations or in refined extracts, include cinchona bark, which contains the chemical quinine that has been used to treat malaria since the 1500s.[3] Years later a secondary effect of this drug was found useful in treating muscle spasms and heart rhythm disturbances. St. John's Wort, which has been used for twenty-five centuries to treat anxiety and depression, [4, 5] in recent years has been found to be as effective as manufactured antidepressants. Foxglove, which is a species of plant that contains the chemical digitoxin, has treated heart disease since the 1400s. [7] It was noted to be a good poison too.

Many think our routine vaccinations are a modern development, yet the Chinese, after much trial and error, performed the first vaccinations for smallpox around 1000 A.D., eight centuries before Western Europeans. By the twentieth century these early principles were followed to produce vaccines for many human scourges, including polio, rabies, diphtheria, tetanus, and influenza.

Caring for the sick was difficult for early American physicians since they had few diagnostic tools, minimal understanding of disease processes, and few effective treatments. If a disease could not be cured by consuming purging agents to empty the bowels, applying mustard plasters to the skin to draw out poisons, lancing boils, or bloodletting, there was no treatment except to allow the human body to heal itself. Sometimes the adverse effects from the treatments outweighed their benefits and were devastating to the patient. One doctor in the 1700s stated, "The harsh treatments punished sick people and could even shorten lives."

The same observation could be made of today's patients who are undergoing chemotherapy for cancer or those patients in our intensive care units who are connected to various machines with tubes coming out of their bodies seemingly from everywhere. Indeed, the lines often become blurred between therapeutic effects and adverse effects of a therapy. The lines of difference change frequently when the discussion concerns babies or the elderly.

Through the years, with all the changes in medical care, both good and bad, and the seemingly endless amount of human suffering, there has been at least one constant. There have been those who were willing to treat the ill and injured with the hope that they could make their patient better. Additionally, the patient had the expectation, warranted or not, that the physician's treatment would cure him. Sometimes the expectations were fulfilled; more often they were not.

This book's title, Side Effects, is meant to hint at the unforeseen events that happen in everyday life and in medicine. Side effects[7] from events or drugs may be considered both positive and negative depending upon the circumstances and one's point of view. Often there exists merely a fine line between a good side effect and a bad one.

Most of the stories deal with unforeseen events; the reader can determine the side effects and if they were good or bad. I have included occasional historical notes or explanations inside the text with the hope that they will enhance the understanding of the story.

This book recounts a few of my experiences from my clinical years. Like my previous books, Reflections of a Country Doctor and The Next Prescription, this book contains stories about real people, my patients, who allowed me the privilege of attending them. Some are silly, some are sad, some are funny, and some may make you mad.

I hope you enjoy sharing this part of my journey.

THE GOOD, THE BAD, THE UGLY

"I do the very best I can, I mean to keep going.
If the end brings me out all right,
then what is said against me won't matter.
If I'm wrong, ten angels swearing I was right
won't make a difference."

Abraham Lincoln

Old Blue Eyes

In the forty years between 1960 and 2000 the amount of research activity in the biomedical fields around the world exploded as pharmaceutical companies spent enormous amounts of money looking for the next blockbuster medical product. In 1985, after thirteen years of intense laboratory experimentation that required the efforts of thousands of employees, Pfizer pharmaceuticals in England produced a compound they hoped would be useful in reducing hypertension (high blood pressure) and treating angina pectoris (chest pain, a symptom of heart disease). The new compound was labeled UK–92480 and was submitted eventually for clinical trials. [8, 9, 10]

Unfortunately, the results for UK-92480 lowering blood pressures were minimal to poor at best. However, this chemical had an interesting side effect in male patients; it produced erections of the penis in almost all the male volunteers. Amazingly, or perhaps not, this drug proved to be surprisingly popular among the male study participants. Even more interesting was the discovery that the drug produced penile erections in patients suffering with diabetes, neurological injuries, and vascular disease who had problems with impotence.

The management at Pfizer realized they had stumbled accidentally across a treatment for erectile dysfunction that could be delivered in a pill form. They had found a blockbuster drug by pure blind luck, and Pfizer had hit the mother load. The chemical was called sildenafil; Pfizer named the product Viagra.

Viagra was packaged as a small blue pill and was introduced to the United States in the spring of 1998. A drug representative first told me about the product in the summer of 1998. At that time, the drug was being promoted for treating males with impotence secondary to medical problems. In particular, Viagra was promoted for patients with diabetes, neurological disease, and premature-onset impotence that had been formally and thoroughly evaluated by a physician. Initially, the drug had no known significant side effects or any adverse reactions when it was taken with other drugs.

One winter day in 1999 I received a call from a nurse in our hospital emergency room. The nurse told me the ambulance crew was attending a male patient in the country who had collapsed in his home. Fortunately, the man did not require cardiopulmonary resuscitation at the time of their evaluations. The ambulance crew requested that I be at the emergency room when they arrived just in case something adverse happened on the way to the hospital. Their estimated arrival time was ten to fifteen minutes.

I got into my pickup promptly and drove to the hospital. I arrived just a few minutes before the ambulance. The nurse was waiting to inform me about the status of the patient. She said the man was in his late fifties and had no blood pressure. She was preparing to perform cardiopulmonary resuscitation when he arrived. The nurse added that the man's wife was coming with him in the ambulance.

As the man was being transferred into the receiving area of the emergency room, the emergency medical technicians (EMTs) were preparing to initiate cardiopulmonary resuscitation (CPR). During my initial examination, however, I noticed that the patient indeed did have a weak pulse and was breathing. Therefore, I asked the EMTs to cease their efforts and transfer the patient to an emergency room bed.

Appearing to be in his late fifties to early sixties, the man had a palpable, faint pulse, and pupils that were reactive and not dilated, which suggested to me that no significant brain injury had occurred. He responded very slowly to a loud voice. I determined his blood pressure to be only about 70 over 50 (normal is 120 over 80), and he had a rapid, irregular, and faint pulse.

First, I started an intravenous catheter for fluids while an electrocardiogram (ECG), an electrical recording of the heart activity, was being performed. The cardiac monitor displayed a regular heart rhythm with some occasional extra beats without any evidence for an acute heart attack. The laboratory technician who was standing by obtained blood samples for testing. Since the man was breathing on his own, he received oxygen applied to his face with a mask. Being cautious, I assigned a nurse to observe his breathing continuously and to have a resuscitation bag nearby ready to assist his breathing as necessary.

Once the ER team had started our patient on all the basic life support procedures and he seemed to be relatively stable for the moment, I turned my attention to the woman who had accompanied the man in the ambulance. Appearing to me to be in her mid-thirties, the woman was wearing merely a robe, house slippers, and a wedding ring. I asked if her husband had any medical problems we should know about.

“No,” the woman replied.

When I asked if her husband took any medications, she replied, “No.”

When I asked her to describe what happened at their home, she said they had been making love most of the day, and all of a sudden, he just collapsed.

After this short discussion, I returned to the emergency room and continued my evaluation of the patient. His cardiac examination was unremarkable except for his low blood pressure and weak pulse. The examination of the man's chest and abdomen was unremarkable. An evaluation of the man's eyes revealed a deep blue coloration of his conjunctiva (the white part), a rather interesting finding. Another peculiar physical finding was that, despite his low blood pressure, the man's penis was erect; a condition called priapism.

About this time, one of the other hospital personnel came up to me and whispered that she was acquainted with our patient’s family. She informed me the woman in the emergency room was not the man's wife.

The patient’s low blood pressure was not responding to the usual treatment of copious intravenous fluids. However, he remained relatively stable and could be awakened. As the emergency room personnel continued to work feverishly to raise our patient’s blood pressure, I took the woman aside and asked her again about what she knew about this man’s medical history.

The woman told me emphatically that I had already asked if her husband had any medical problems, and she repeated that her husband did not have any medical problems nor did he did not take any medicines. The woman then expressed to me firmly and pointedly that the man I was treating was not her husband; he was her lover.

I asked if she knew where the man's real wife was.

She revealed to me that the wife was on a two-week vacation in Hawaii and added her husband was on an educational trip to Acapulco learning about ranching.

I questioned the woman again if she knew if our patient, her lover, had any medical issues.

The woman replied that, although she did not know of any for sure, he had been taking pills to make himself perform better in bed.

When I asked how many pills the man had taken, she

informed me they had been having sex somewhere between three and six times a day for the past week. She assumed her lover was taking a pill to give himself an erection each time they had sex, and she added, "He didn't want to disappoint me, you know."

The woman also noted that just before he collapsed, the man said he was feeling funny. She saw him take a little tablet and put it under his tongue thinking it was just taking another pill for her lover to perform better in bed.

When I asked if she saw what the pill looked like or what kind of bottle it was in, the woman admitted she did not see the pill. However, she noticed that her boyfriend took the pill from a small dark bottle.

This description made me think the man took a nitroglycerin pill for a cardiac condition since these pills are packaged in small dark bottles to prevent deterioration from light.

The man's physical findings and clinical presentation suggested to me that he had suffered an adverse reaction to Viagra. Blue conjunctiva was well documented in the medical literature as a sign for having had an overdose of the medication. Some men thought that if one pill was good and two were better, then a bunch would be fantastic. Unfortunately, most medications do not work this way, especially Viagra.

Additionally, he had an erect penis while his blood pressure was quite low. This also suggested that he was having extended and adverse effects from the Viagra.

Finally, the man's heart rhythm disturbance, when coupled with his history and other physical findings, suggested to me that he was having additional adverse side effects from a Viagra overdose.

After a short discussion with the nurses, we raised the man's legs above the level of his heart so all the blood from his legs would drain into his main vascular system. This maneuver was intended to help fill the man's vascular system without adding more fluids intravenously. After several hours and many liters of intravenous fluids, our patient's blood pressure stabilized to near normal, his heart rhythm improved but was not normal yet, and he started to wake up. His mental function was slow but operative. The priapism resolved too. Thereafter, the nurses transported him to our intensive care unit for further observation.

The man remained in our hospital for several days recuperating. During that time, I determined that he had been fortunate indeed. He had not suffered a heart attack or a stroke, nor had he died. I also learned from my patient that his cardiologist in a nearby city had given him prescriptions for both Viagra and nitroglycerin tablets at the same visit. I figured the cardiologist had missed the latest medical bulletins and the many television commercial warnings about using Viagra in patients with heart disease and taking nitroglycerin. I took the liberty of sending the doctor our hospital records of his patient's medical misadventure.

I never met or heard from the gentleman, his girlfriend, or his physician after he left our hospital. I always wondered how he explained the hospital bill to his wife.

With time, more adverse side effect reports emerged from the use of Viagra. These were followed by extensive package insert warnings regarding its proper use. In particular, the use of Viagra by people with significant heart disease, especially those patients taking nitroglycerin and high blood pressure medications, was not recommended. Strokes, heart attacks, heart rhythm disturbances, and deaths were reported. Bizarre hearing and eye disorders and multiple unusual side effects also emerged. [11, 12]

For those young men who wanted to impress women with their sexual stamina, the drug was found not to work very well in young, healthy men without an organic reason for erectile dysfunction.

In the ensuing years, despite the many precautions for its use, Viagra, the little blue pill, became one of the most widely recognized brands in the world and started a sexual revolution worldwide. The "age related male impotence disorder" of my medical school years was transformed into the disease of "Erectile Dysfunction Disorder" which later became known as the "Male Sexual Dysfunction Disorder." Famous politicians and celebrities appeared in television, radio, and newsprint advertising promoting Viagra. Its worldwide sales topped one billion dollars yearly, and it became, and remains, one of Pfizer Corporation's highest grossing prescription drugs ever.

One Hairy Adventure

On a late spring day in 1978 a middle-aged divorced woman named Anna came into my office. Her young adult daughter whom I had seen previously in my clinic as a patient escorted her. Anna was having difficulty controlling her blood pressure, and the daughter thought I could provide a second opinion for her mother.

A cardiologist physician in a nearby city in North Dakota was caring for Anna. Reportedly, she was already taking three different medications, and her blood pressure was not yet controlled. Anna asked me to evaluate her medications and to make some recommendations.

I was a bit bewildered by her request since I thought the cardiologist surely would be able to manage this woman's blood pressure. Despite my uncertainty, I assured Anna and her daughter I would do my best.

I asked Anna if she had brought any of her medical records from her cardiologist. She denied that she had any of her medical records. Consequently, I asked Anna to return to the clinic later in the afternoon after I had an opportunity to call her doctor's office for her medical records. Anna and her daughter agreed to return in the afternoon.

I called the physician's office in North Dakota and identified myself as a physician to the doctor's nurse who answered the phone. To expedite the information transfer, I requested a verbal response for any laboratory or x-ray tests that Anna's physician had obtained. Much to my surprise, the nurse revealed that her physician had not obtained any type of laboratory data for the patient. He had been seeing Anna for almost a year and had not obtained any basic testing that usually was performed before any medication was given for high blood pressure. In my view, this woman should have had at least testing regarding her blood electrolytes, her kidney function, and possibly some x-rays to determine any structural abnormalities of her kidneys.

I thanked the nurse for her time and waited for Anna and her daughter.

The women returned to my office that afternoon as they had promised, and I informed them that her physician in North Dakota had not obtained any blood, urine, or x-ray data to evaluate the possible causes for her hypertension. Anna confirmed that no tests had ever been done.

I explained to them that this seemed a little bit irregular to me.

I took my new patient's blood pressure. Despite her three medications, the blood pressure remained well above normal.

I suggested to Anna that I should obtain some basic laboratory and x-ray tests to help me determine the cause of her severe hypertension. She thought the tests would be a good idea.

During further discussions in my office, Anna and her daughter revealed that they would be traveling to Oregon in a few weeks to visit relatives and that they would be in the Portland area for about two to three months during the summer.

I informed the pair that I had graduated from the University of Oregon Medical School in Portland, Oregon. Instead of my obtaining laboratory tests and playing with the medications for her severe hypertension, I suggested that Anna could be evaluated more thoroughly by the world-class doctors at the University of Oregon Medical School who specialized in kidney diseases and hypertension. Anna thought this was a marvelous idea, and visiting with the Oregon doctors would fit right into her plans.

I asked Anna to give me the dates she was going to be in Oregon. I told Anna that I would arrange for her to be seen at the medical school clinic soon after her arrival in Oregon and requested that she call or come to the clinic the next day so I could give her the specifics for the doctor's appointment.

After they left the clinic, I called the Department of Nephrology (diseases of the kidney) at the University of Oregon Medical School that was headed by Dr. Will Benjamin, M.D. and arranged an appointment for her to be seen in the medical clinic by Dr. Benjamin's team soon after her arrival in Portland.

When Anna returned to see me the next day, I reported my discussions with the people at the medical school. I gave her the names, phone numbers, and places to go at the University and drew her a diagram on how to get to the clinic. Finally, I asked her to continue on her same three medications until she saw the doctors in Oregon.

About three months later in late summer, Anna and her daughter came back to see me in the clinic. Anna, who was crying and most distraught, reported that she had visited the University medical school as arranged. She saw many doctors in the department of kidney diseases where they spent about eight weeks getting her medications straightened out and her blood pressure stabilized. Besides her previous three medications, the doctors at the medical school found that her blood pressure stabilized nicely after adding a brand new blood pressure medication called Loniten. [13, 14, 15]

Anna continued to tell me that a few days after she returned to northeastern Montana, she and her daughter went to visit the cardiologist in North Dakota. She apparently gave the physician her story about visiting the doctors at the University of Oregon Medical School, the testing they did, and the medications she was taking. Anna also presented him with a copy of their records and the results of the testing they had done. Anna told me the doctor picked up her medicines and threw them into the garbage saying that those university doctors were quacks and the medicines they prescribed were going to kill her.

After verifying her mother's story, the daughter stated the cardiologist wrote her mother four new prescriptions for blood pressure medications.

Obviously, both of the women were quite shocked over this incident. They had come to me again for another opinion.

After reading the medical records from the University physicians, I asked Anna if she had the prescriptions with her. She related that she had filled the four prescriptions ordered by the cardiologist. The daughter interjected that she had retrieved the four medications from the garbage and brought them to show me.

I compared the medications and determined the cardiologist had prescribed exactly the same four medications that the doctors in Oregon had prescribed. The doctors in Oregon had used the generic names for the medication labels while the cardiologist used the trade names for the prescription labels, so I explained to the women that the two sets of medications were identical.

Anna was incredulous and confused while her daughter asked me why the cardiologist would act that way toward her mother.

I could say only that I did not know. I then took out a medication book called the Physicians Desk Reference (PDR) and showed the women the pages where it displayed the generic medicines being exactly the same as the proprietary medicines. I put the pills side-by-side and showed them that the two sets of medications were identical.

Again, the daughter asked why the cardiologist would do such a thing. Again, I had no explanation.

Once I had convinced Anna and her daughter the medications

were the same, they wondered if it would be all right if Anna continued to see me for her blood pressure medications instead of the cardiologist. I agreed to continue caring for Anna.

Following the requests of the physicians in Oregon, I checked Anna's blood pressure weekly, and it remained quite stable over the next several months. However, Anna started to complain that she was becoming very hairy in places where she should not have hair. In particular, she was developing eyebrows that were almost touching between her eyes, sideburns, very hairy legs, hair on her chest, and a mustache with a beard.

I reviewed the literature for her medications at the time and no such side effects were identified. I thought the phenomenon must be a side effect of the four different medicines used together.

About this time, Anna revealed to me that she and her daughter would be returning to Oregon to visit family during the Thanksgiving holiday season. I suggested they revisit the University of Oregon physicians to see what they had to say about her hairiness.

The women thought this to be an excellent plan.

Anna returned to see me again several months later just after the New Year. She said the doctors at the University of Oregon Medical School thought she was having an adverse side effect from Loniten and advised her that a few people had developed severe unwanted hair growth from that medication. Subsequently, her Loniten was discontinued, and another medication was substituted for it. Anna also mentioned that the doctors in Oregon informed her about reports that were emerging which connected the drug to many severe side effects, such as patients dying abruptly, heart failure, heart attacks, heart rhythm disorders, strokes, and other serious maladies. Therefore, the doctors were more than happy to stop the drug.

At this visit, Anna was happy. All the unwanted hair on her head, face, and legs was gone. The blood pressure was normal, and her new medications seemed to be keeping her blood pressure in good control. When she left the university, all of her blood and kidney tests were reported as normal.

I wrote a follow-up letter to the doctors at the University of Oregon Medical School and related my patient's good follow-up blood pressure control and hair loss results.

Soon thereafter I received a call from one of the medical residents at the University. He informed me that Loniten had been discontinued at the University because of its severe side effect profile. Additionally, he told me they found the side effect of hypertrichosis, or excessive hair growth, to be annoying to many patients, especially women.

Loniten has a generic name of minoxidil and never achieved much success as a blood pressure drug. In some types of patients, the drug became infamous for its severe adverse side effects.

One particular extreme adverse effect of the minoxidil that did not go unnoticed by the manufacturer, Upjohn Pharmaceuticals, was the unexplained excessive hair proliferation. In the late 1970s the minoxidil was reformulated and diverted into clinical trials that specifically investigated hair growth stimulation in men. By 1986 a dilute solution of minoxidil, marketed as Rogaine, was made available in the United States.

It has never been determined exactly how minoxidil causes hair to grow, but the medication when prepared in a dilute solution is effective in reversing male pattern hair loss in many men and women and has no major side effects. [16, 17, 18, 19]

Rogaine for hair loss produced a revolution in hair loss therapy for men and eventually for women. It became one of the most recognized drugs in history and remains the leading treatment for hair loss worldwide. For the Upjohn Company, minoxidil ascended from Loniten, a blood pressure drug catastrophe, to Rogaine, a worldwide hair-raising success.

More Than Meets the Eye

I became acquainted with Burrell just after I arrived in Sidney in 1976. Within a few months after my arrival, Burrell's family physician moved away, and he allowed me the privilege of assuming his care.

Burrell, a portly middle-aged man, had a multitude of problems. He had a long-term history of allergies and asthma since childhood that were exacerbated by his smoking a pipe and by the seasonal air pollution in our valley associated with the local agriculture industry and sugar beet refining. In addition, he had developed early onset cataracts, which resulted in their surgical removal some years before. This was done in the era before the development of artificial lens implants when there were no lens substitutes to replace the removed cataracts in the eye. Associated with his eye disease was glaucoma, which is an elevation of the pressure within the eye itself.

Burrell's allergies and asthma were usually controlled with a variety of medications. His eye pressure was, for the most part, controlled with a combination of several different glaucoma medications that were commonly prescribed at the time by ophthalmologists who are physician specialists in eye diseases.

My early examinations of Burrell revealed evidence of chronic obstructive pulmonary disease (COPD) and asthma that was moderately severe. He also had moderately severe high blood pressure. Examinations of his nose revealed evidence of chronic allergies.

Since he lived in an area with considerable agricultural air pollutants, an arid environment, and factories, Burrell had learned how "to just get by" with his asthma and his allergies. However, his symptoms were never well controlled. He informed me that several times yearly he required injections of cortisone when his symptoms became very bad. His records from his previous local physicians and an allergy specialist confirmed this history.

In early January of 1979, Burrell met me in the hospital and told me his usual asthma medications were not working. He was having increasing difficulty breathing, particularly during the night, and his exercise tolerance was down to nil. He denied any recent infections, and it was in the middle of winter when his allergy symptoms were usually the best. Burrell was a bit perplexed why he was having so much trouble.

I asked Burrell to intensify his treatments for asthma and COPD and gave him instructions how to do it.

A short time later, Burrell talked with me outside of my clinic. He said his ophthalmologist had recently given him a brand-new medicine for his glaucoma called Timoptic. [20, 21] He related that his doctor told him the medicine was essentially without side effects and should do wonders for his eye pressure control. In addition, he had to take the medicine only twice a day instead of the every four hours dosing that was required by his current regimen of several medications. Burrell asked me if his new medication could be causing his increased trouble with breathing.

I related to him that the drug was new and I knew nothing about it, but I would further research it. I suggested that we could perform some lung function testing on him in my clinic to determine if the new medicine was making his asthma worse.

Burrell thought this was a reasonable idea.

We arranged to meet in the clinic the next day to discuss my research findings and to perform pulmonary function tests for his asthma I planned to perform the test both before and after Burrell took his new eye medication.

We met the next morning as arranged. I told him I had talked with the hospital's pharmacist, and the information I could find on his new medication was similar to what his physician had already given him. That is, as far as the drug company knew, or at least reported, the medication was without any significant complications or adverse side effects.

Timoptic (generic name is timolol) is in a class of drugs called nonspecific beta-blocker (ß blocker) that was developed mostly to control high blood pressure and to treat heart disease. These blood pressure drugs, which were in pill form and at much higher doses, were well known to cause problems with asthma and emphysema patients. Timoptic was prepared in an eye drop solution and contained only a fraction of the medication found in the pills.

I had Burrell perform a pulmonary function test by blowing into a special device that recorded the amount of air he could blow out and the speed with which he could expel the air from his lungs. The test revealed that his asthma and his COPD were about as good as usual. I then placed a single drop of his new medication into just one of his eyes. Within about a minute, Burrell noted he was not feeling very good. A repeat pulmonary function test revealed essentially no airflow in his lungs. He could not breathe.

Burrell collapsed immediately and fell to the floor. He lost consciousness.

Immediately, I called out to my nurse for assistance and gave him an emergency injection of adrenalin, which is a powerful airway dilator medication. A similar medication was given through his mouth by way of a nebulizer and a mask. Fortunately, within a matter of seconds Burrell awakened and started to breathe better.

After another fifteen minutes, when I assured myself that Burrell was stable and coherent, I explained to him what had happened. I advised that he should no longer take his new glaucoma medicine and suggested he restart his old glaucoma medicine regimen and await further instructions from his ophthalmologist. Furthermore, I told Burrell that I would send a copy of my office notes to his ophthalmologist and to the Food and Drug Administration (FDA) to report an observed adverse drug event. Finally, I told him I would send a copy of his records to a doctor at the University of Washington School of Medicine in Seattle, Washington, who had done some of the studies on this medication.

Burrell's ophthalmologist, after receiving the medical records, promptly took him off the new medication and restarted his old glaucoma regimen using multiple medications. Afterward his glaucoma control returned to its normal steady state and so did his asthma.

Several months later I had a telephone conversation with my father-in-law who had a similar history to Burrell's of having had early onset cataracts with associated glaucoma after eye surgery. He too was on the old regimen of several drugs to control his eye pressure, and he too had mild asthma according to his physician. My father-in-law said he had just started a wonderful new medicine for his glaucoma that did not burn his eyes, he had to use it only once a day, and he did not have blurred vision after he took the medicine. Later in the conversation he divulged to me that he was having an awful lot of trouble sleeping at night because of coughing.

I asked him if he was having trouble breathing at night.

He didn't think so. He just was coughing all night.

I knew that coughing at night was a classic sign for asthma. I asked my father-in-law if he knew the name of the eye drops.

After he found the bottle, he said the name on the bottle was Timoptic and then spelled the name for me.

I suggested that the reason for his coughing might be asthma, which was being produced by this new glaucoma medicine. I told him I would call Dr. Hargrave, his ophthalmologist in Billings, Montana, and relate our discussion. Afterward he and Dr. Hargrave could further discuss the treatment for his glaucoma.

I telephoned Dr. Hargrave, and after I related my father-in-law's story to him, he replied, "I was just at a meeting in Southern California. There was considerable talk about Timoptic and its side effects with asthma, lung disease, and heart attacks. They told us that glaucoma patients with heart and lung problems were dropping like flies in Southern California." He then said he would call my father-in-law as soon as he got off the telephone with me and have him restart his old glaucoma therapy.

I talked with my father-in-law about a week later and asked him if he was still coughing all night. He expressed relief that the coughing ended the day after he stopped the Timoptic eye drops. He reported that Dr. Hargrave advised him never to take any beta-blocker medication again.

Before 1978, our anti-glaucoma medical treatment options included three or four different classes of drugs used simultaneously. Unfortunately, significant problems attended the use of all these medications. By eliminating many of the side effects of these drugs, which included blurred vision, facial pain, redness of the eyes, eye discomfort upon administration, rashes, kidney stones, and a host of other problems, and by reducing the dosing frequency from every three to four hours for each medicine to once or twice a day for a single medicine, timolol (Timoptic) soon became the most popular first drug used by ophthalmologists worldwide for the medical treatment of glaucoma.

Although initial reports described timolol as highly safe and effective, clinical experience and long term studies exposed a long list of its potential adverse effects in certain groups of individuals which included a slow heart rate, heart rhythm disturbances, congestive heart failure, and syncope in heart patients, worsening of asthma and COPD in lung patients, and a wide range of problems from depression to hair loss. Between 1978 and 1980, four hundred fifty cases of severe heart and lung events attributed to Timoptic were reported to the FDA (Food and Drug Administration) with thirty-two deaths reported. The FDA estimates that only one adverse drug event for every one thousand that occurs is ever reported. Therefore, Timoptic harmed potentially thousands more people.

In time, increased knowledge of this drug's limitations and adverse effects allowed ophthalmologists to select more accurately the patients who could be treated, or, what was more important, who should not be treated with beta-blockers for glaucoma.

Burrell continued with his older type glaucoma medication regimen until the early 1990s. By now, his eye physician had retired, and his new ophthalmologist wanted to try another new glaucoma medicine that was similar to the one that gave Burrell trouble years before but supposedly had far fewer side effects. The doctor gave Burrell a small sample bottle as a trial. Being a bit wary, Burrell promptly informed me of this medication change for his glaucoma.

After a short discussion, we decided to test Burrell's lung function as we had done before and arrangements were made in the clinic for the testing to be done. Again, I had Burrell perform a breathing function test before and after receiving the new medication into only one eye. As before, Burrell's lung function dropped substantially after receiving merely a single drop of the new medication. His pulmonary function did not completely collapse as it had done the first time, but his lung function diminished by at least fifty percent. This time I was able to restore Burrell's lung function to its baseline state with the simple administration of medication through an aerosol nebulizer for about an hour.

I showed Burrell the paper recording of his lung function tests and how the test results worsened after just one drop of medication. I suggested he return to his original medication regimen for his glaucoma. He smiled and said it was worth a try because he knew I was protecting him.

I sent a copy of the records to his new ophthalmologist that afternoon. Additionally, I called the ophthalmologist soon after the test to inform him of the results.

The ophthalmologist told me had he was assured by the drug representatives that this new drug did not have the significant side effects of the beta-blocker class of drugs, particularly Timoptic. He said he would telephone Burrell at home that evening to see how he was doing. The ophthalmologist mentioned to me that he would put a note in Burrell's chart that stated he "should no longer and forevermore NOT take a beta blocker medication for any reason!"

It turned out the new drug was nothing more than a slightly

modified Timoptic.

Timolol was marketed initially as a blood pressure reduction medication named Blocadren, which proved to be not very effective when compared to similar drugs. However, for some unknown reason and despite its side effects, timolol as a glaucoma treatment was different and a major improvement from all the other medications used to treat glaucoma. In the more than twenty-five years since its introduction, timolol (Timoptic) has been nothing but gold. It remains the gold standard worldwide for the initial treatment of glaucoma for many patients. [22, 23]

My father-in-law and Burrell, who were two exceptions to this gold standard, never used Timoptic or any other beta-blocker medication again.

Bad Medicine

In May 1979 the SmithKline pharmaceutical company marketed a new type of diuretic medication named Selacryn. [24] The drug had been used in Europe for almost two decades before it was finally approved for use in United States. Most diuretic medications, besides making a patient urinate more often, make a patient's kidneys lose potassium and magnesium through the urine and increase the blood level of a chemical called uric acid. This is particularly troublesome in patients who have gout, a disorder with an excess of the chemical uric acid in the blood and joints. Selacryn did none of these things. It was promoted for those patients who needed diuretic medications and who had difficulty with high uric acid levels and low potassium levels in the blood.

I was introduced to this medication in June 1979. Soon after the drug representative gave me the literature about this new medication, I knew I had several patients with gouty arthritis who might benefit from its use.

I discussed Selacryn with some kidney and arthritis specialists in a nearby referral center and found out that they too were excited about using this new drug.

One of my patients afflicted with gouty arthritis who required a diuretic for another medical problem was Marjorie Danskin. Soon after I learned about Selacryn, I had the opportunity to visit with Marjorie in my clinic. After I had discussed the medication with her, she was agreeable to see if it worked for her.

Subsequently, I gave Marjorie a sample supply of Selacryn to last several weeks to determine if she could tolerate it. If she had any difficulties with the new medication, Marjorie was to notify me promptly. Otherwise, I asked her to return to see me in several weeks. When she returned, I planned to do some blood tests to see if her blood uric acid and potassium levels remained stable, increased, or decreased. My hope was that the uric acid levels would decrease and the potassium levels would remain stable or increase.

Marjorie returned several weeks later as I had requested and had her blood tests. The medication worked as advertised. Not only did Marjorie get the diuretic effect of the medication, but also her uric acid level decreased which made her gout symptoms less. Her potassium and magnesium levels remained stable without further supplementation with minerals. To say the least, we were both quite excited with the results of this new drug.

I gave Marjorie a prescription for six months, and she promised to see me in three months to make sure all was going well.

At her three-month visit Marjorie was indeed doing well. Instead of taking four pills a day as she had done before, she was only taking a single pill, Selacryn. I was impressed with the results and asked Marjorie to continue on the medication for another year. However, I asked her to see me again in another six months for more blood tests. I encouraged Marjorie to contact me promptly if she did not feel well in any way during the next six months.

I did not see Marjorie until the fall of the next year when she came to our hospital emergency room. Her skin was bright orange, she had severe upper abdominal pain, and she had lost a considerable amount of weight. Marjorie was emaciated and appeared to me like she was dying. When I asked where she had been since her last visit, she admitted that she had decided to see another doctor for her care. I told her I had no problem with her changing physicians. I asked her the name of her current physician so I could contact him about her illness.

Marjorie said that she had been seeing a natural physician in North Dakota who had been treating her illnesses naturally with daily colonics or enemas, nutritional supplements, and a vegetarian diet.

When I asked about her high uric acid levels and her gout, Marjorie said her natural physician told her that she never had those problems. He convinced Marjorie her previous physicians, including me, were quacks.

When I asked her about the problems that required her to use a diuretic, Marjorie said she didn't need the medicine after she started taking daily colonics and drinking less water.

When I inquired about the yellow color of her skin, Marjorie said her natural doctor assured her that it was related to her eating large quantities of yellow vegetables; the yellow tint of her skin supposedly was the pigment from the vegetables and was not a major concern.

When I questioned her about why she came to the emergency room on this particular day, Marjorie revealed to me that morning was the worst she had felt in a very long time. Apparently she'd not been feeling well for several months and was hoping the treatments given to her by the naturalist physician would cure her. Finally her husband insisted she go to see a real doctor in the hospital, and I just happened to be the physician on call in the emergency room.

Marjorie's blood tests returned and revealed her uric acid level was much higher than I had ever seen it, and her potassium level was critically low. All of her liver enzymes were markedly elevated, suggesting some type of hepatitis or other activity in her liver. Her complete blood count showed all the test results to be extremely low, suggesting that Marjorie's body was being overwhelmed by an infection or something much worse, like a cancerous tumor.

A physical examination of Marjorie's abdomen revealed considerable tenderness under her right rib cage. Masses that I thought were her liver were large, hard, and exquisitely tender to light touch. She also had enlarged lymph nodes under her arms and in her groin.

I ordered a computerized scan (CT) of her abdomen which revealed an enlarged liver with multiple masses within it as well as other tumor areas throughout her abdomen and chest. Her yellow skin was a direct consequence of her liver ducts being obstructed by the tumors and her liver being destroyed.

I became frustrated with what I saw because this woman's naturalist physician had missed a bad problem. In my opinion, Marjorie was suffering the consequences of this person's neglect.

Marjorie was admitted into the hospital, and I obtained consultations from the local surgeon and two internal medicine specialists. They all agreed that no treatment would be beneficial at this late stage of advanced liver cancer.

I introduced Marjorie to the nurses of the hospice program in our community. When she left our hospital to go to her home a few days later, Marjorie received full-time nursing and hospice care. She died at her home a just few days later. Marjorie was just forty-five years old.

The SmithKline pharmaceutical company removed Selacryn from the market in the spring of 1980 after being on the market for less than a year. In that short time in the United States market, it was determined that this drug had a major adverse side effect of acute hepatitis and liver cancer. Despite the glowing reports in the pharmacy literature, the promotional literature given to physicians, and the drug's package inserts, the details of the hepatitis and cancer complications that had become apparent years before during clinical trials and years before the drug was first released were not revealed until after the drug was removed from the marketplace.

The pharmaceutical company had lied, and they got caught.

Between 1980 and 1984 the SmithKline Company paid out millions of dollars in compensation to victims of Selacryn. In 1984, the SmithKline Company and its three top medical executives pleaded guilty to over thirty counts of misconduct relating to this drug.[25]

After Marjorie died, I wondered how much of her serious illness was caused by the actions, or inactions, of her naturalist physician. I wondered what role Selacryn had contributed to her suffering and if it was the cause. Could I have used another therapy to help her?

I still wonder.

Jump Start

In the late 1980s Tim came to visit me in my clinic. As I entered the examination room, Tim exclaimed, "Doc, have I got a story for you," and went on to tell me about playing in a charity golf tournament in Billings, Montana, several weeks before. Tim said he was on the tenth tee box when, while making his backswing to tee off, it felt like something hit him in the chest and dropped him like a rock. He continued to tell me he lost consciousness and woke up in the hospital emergency room hooked up to all sorts of monitors with an intravenous catheter in his arm and surrounded by a group of people in white coats.

One of the people standing around him who appeared to be the doctor in charge informed Tim that he had almost died. The doctor went on to tell Tim and his wife that he had experienced a dangerous heart rhythm disturbance on the golf course during which his heart essentially stopped beating correctly causing him to collapse. It was Tim's good fortune that his fellow golfers started cardiopulmonary resuscitation (CPR) on him on the tee box. Tim was later informed that when the ambulance arrived, the EMTs gave him some medicine in a vein that stabilized his heart rhythm. After he arrived in the emergency room, his abnormal rhythm returned, and the hospital personnel had to shock him several times before his normal heart rhythm returned.

Tim related that he spent the next week or so in the hospital during which the cardiologist offered him either a pacemaker or some medication to keep his heart rhythm stable for the rest of his days. If he did neither, the doctor informed him the next episode could be fatal.

Tim said he told the cardiologist that he was not really keen on having a battery and some booster cables in his chest to zap him whenever his heart rate became irregular. Since the doctor apparently encouraged him to take some medicine, Tim decided to take the prescription pills. Tim explained that he was in the office just for a checkup at the request of his cardiologist.

I knew that Tim, who was in his late fifties, had been in excellent health before this episode. He was an avid outdoorsman who loved to snow ski, hike, play sports, and hunt. He walked or ran every day and never smoked cigarettes. Only occasionally did he consume an alcoholic drink. All the men in his family had lived until their ninth decade.

I related to Tim that it sounded to me like he was a pretty lucky fellow. He just smiled and nodded yes. I asked if he had been having any difficulties from a physical standpoint since he left the hospital. Tim confessed that he seemed to be tired and lacked energy but assumed this was a result of his medical incident. He remained unable to perform physically as well as he had before.

When I asked if he could be more specific with things that were bothering him, Tim responded that he couldn't put his finger on any one thing.

Even though I continued my normal history taking with Tim, he offered no more positive answers to my questions. During my physical examination I noticed that Tim's heart rate thankfully was regular. When I listened to his lungs, I heard wheezing throughout his chest. After I asked Tim again if he ever had any difficulties with allergies or asthma, he insisted he never had any allergies to medicines and never had asthma.

I performed a lung function test which revealed his lung function to be diminished by about thirty percent. This decrease in lung function could not be improved by my giving Tim medications to open up his airways. Therefore, I knew his wheezing was caused by something other than asthma. I told Tim that I needed to get an x-ray of his chest to see what was going on in his lungs and sent him to radiology.

The chest x-ray revealed a generalized process in both lungs that had a ground glass appearance similar to that I had seen many times in premature newborn babies with breathing problems. I advised Tim of my findings and told him I was going to call his cardiologist in Billings, Montana, right away. While Tim waited in the examination room, I telephoned his cardiologist and relayed my findings.

This cardiologist was concerned that Tim was having an adverse reaction to his new medication, which was called amiodarone, [26, 27] and wanted him to come to Billings immediately.

I gave this information to Tim who telephoned his wife promptly. He asked her to pack a travel bag, make a few phone calls, and plan on going to Billings for an unknown period of time. After perhaps half an hour she arrived at my office, and the pair started their journey to Billings.

That evening, I obtained some information from the local pharmacy and our medical library about amiodarone. Its history of becoming a usable drug was quite interesting.

Amiodarone, which was marketed as Pacerone, has a parent chemical compound called khellin that comes from the khella plant, which is common in North Africa. Apparently, a Lebanese researcher working in Cairo, Egypt, in the 1950s noticed one of his African assistants had been cured of his cardiac pain (angina) after taking khellin. Native Africans also used this plant for a variety of other non-cardiac ailments. The amiodarone compound itself was initially developed in the early 1960s by chemists in Belgium.

As biochemical evaluations of the chemical continued over the next decade, it was determined that, besides it's anti-angina properties, it possessed properties that could modify heart rhythm disturbances.

By the early 1980s the drug was commonly prescribed in Europe and in South America for patients with life threatening heart rhythm disturbances. The experience during this initial use of amiodarone allowed physicians time to acknowledge its extensive severe adverse side effect profile. In particular, amiodarone produced serious pulmonary problems in literally hundreds of patients which resulted in many having severe disabilities and many deaths.

During the drug's early years, the American Food and Drug Administration (FDA) did not allow it to be sold here because of its poor adverse side effect profile. Apparently because of political pressures in America and abroad, the FDA finally approved amiodarone in December 1985 for the treatment of severe cardiac rhythm disturbances. This made amiodarone one of just a few drugs the FDA has ever approved without any rigorous controlled randomized clinical testing. (Unfortunately, this statement also includes most psychiatric drugs.)

One of the primary adverse side effects of Pacerone is a severe hypersensitivity reaction, and there is no known antidote for the drug or for this complication. Since the drug stays in the body up to four months, whatever hypersensitivity reaction occurs will be maintained for that length of time until the body eliminates it naturally.

I received a call from Tim's cardiologist a day or so later who informed me that Tim apparently had an acute pulmonary hypersensitivity reaction to the amiodarone. The cardiologist had referred him to a team of lung disease specialists called pulmonologists to care for him. Unfortunately, none of the doctors had seen this complication of amiodarone before and were not sure exactly how to treat it.

Tim came to my office about six months later. Because he had been given massive doses of cortisone[28, 29] to slow down the allergy reaction in his lungs, he had gained about thirty pounds, and his entire body was bloated. Additionally, when the medication was stopped, Tim's life-threatening heart rhythm disturbances returned, and the cardiologist was compelled to insert a pacemaker into Tim's heart to keep him alive.

Tim was quite short of breath, and his exercise tolerance was minimal. He had difficulty walking just a few feet before he had to sit down. His wife informed me that the doctors in Billings did not know when or if Tim would regain his strength. The damage to his lungs had been substantial and now, during the healing phase of his injury, his lungs were scarring down. She said the pulmonologist called the disorder pulmonary fibrosis.

To compound the problems, the cardiologist informed them that the amiodarone was responsible for damaging Tim's heart even more. Now he took two heart medicines to complement his pacemaker.

Over the next five years, Tim slowly improved, but, unfortunately, his lung function remained drastically reduced. Although he no longer could walk the golf course, Tim could play now if he rode in a cart. He gave up skiing, hiking, and hunting. Tim became deeply depressed for which he received professional counseling and more medications. Tim and his wife also moved to be closer to his many doctors.

The couple learned about the well known severe adverse effects of the drug some time after he first received it. The doctor who originally encouraged him to take the drug never presented the facts that severe pulmonary side effects occurred in up to fifteen percent of the patients taking it. A legal challenge to the doctor and the pharmaceutical company settled out of court in Tim's favor.

Despite its severe side effect profile, amiodarone not only became a favorite drug of the cardiology community worldwide but also gained a primary recommendation in cardiac emergency protocols for ACLS programs (Advanced Cardiac Life Support) by the American Heart Association.

I, however, refused to use the drug. I taught the ACLS course in our region of Montana for more than two decades; I always explained to my students why I refused to use amiodarone even though it was recommended. Other older drugs were just as effective for heart rhythm disturbances in my view without the potential for the drastic sequelae of amiodarone.

I met Tim downtown about ten years after his original heart episode. He was now in his late sixties and in Sidney visiting some friends. He informed me he was mostly homebound except for a few outside activities that required minimal physical activity. He lamented that he was just getting by.

Sometime later I wondered what would have happened to Tim years before if he had chosen the battery and booster cables instead of the pill.

Too Many Pills

At least once per month over my thirty plus years in family practice, I would have a patient come into my clinic with a curious assortment of maladies. All too often these patients had been seen previously by a collection of specialist physicians who had not communicated well with each other about their mutual patient. Consequently, the patient arrived at my office confused, often misinformed, feeling neglected, and still not feeling well. The patient, or a family member, usually would ask me to help them sort out and explain their problems.

Through the years I taught medical students and family medicine residents that our American medical care system was so disjointed that there needed to be quarterbacks for the healthcare team. I saw my job as one of these quarterbacks who tried to educate his patients and tried to make sense of what my patient's collective team of specialists was trying to accomplish.

A classic example of the dilemmas I experienced was the case of seventy-year-old Marshall Ballard who asked me just to review his medications. This man had been referred to me by another one of my patients whom I had helped evaluate his medications. Mr. Ballard complained that he just didn't feel good.

Mr. Ballard lived near Sidney and, while visiting friends in Washington State about six weeks before, had an episode in which he suddenly felt very tired and could not move from his chair. His family members rushed him to the emergency room at a local hospital where doctors determined Marshall had suffered a very small heart attack.

Before he knew it, Marshall was in a special room where a cardiologist put stents into two of his heart arteries. The next morning while he was recovering, Marshall was given what he called a handful of pills. Before this episode, Marshall related he seldom, if ever, took a pill for anything and, therefore, was what some physicians would call a medication virgin.

There was no way the doctors could determine Marshall's tolerance to any single medication by giving him a handful of pills at a time. Medications, especially when administered to patients over sixty years old, should be given with a very small starting dose, and the doses should be increased gradually over time until the desired therapeutic effect is attained. Unfortunately for Marshall, this process was not done because it requires several weeks' time with close monitoring of the patient, and most physicians do not have or take the necessary time or have the needed resources to devote to each patient.

Marshall reported to me that he remained in Washington for two weeks and was referred to a cardiologist in Billings, Montana, for follow-up care and cardiac rehabilitation.

Marshall handed me his medication bottles to examine. They included medicines to slow down his heart rate, to thin his blood, to reduce the level of cholesterol in his blood, and to make him sleep.

After having taken all these medicines for a couple weeks, I asked Marshall how he felt. He said he absolutely had no energy, but the doctors assured him the fatigue was a result of his heart attack and that he should get his strength back in a few weeks.

Furthermore, Marshall told me that during the same time after his heart attack his memory went to hell, his muscles ached all over his body, especially in his legs, and, despite taking the sleeping pill, he was awake all night. He said he felt drunk all the time.

Marshall apparently told the cardiologist in Billings and his associate about his problems, but he noted they dismissed the idea that his problems were caused by the medications. Instead, the cardiologist referred him to a neurologist for his memory issues.

Reportedly, the neurologist could not see Marshall that day, and his physician assistant, without performing a physical examination, referred him in turn to an orthopedic surgeon to evaluate his muscle aches. Marshall said the orthopedic surgeon worked him into his clinic schedule that day.

When Marshall described his muscle aches, which were worst in his legs, the orthopedist sent him to have an MRI scan of his back before he even examined him. When the MRI scan did not divulge anything the orthopedist could fix surgically, Marshall was returned to the neurologist to evaluate his muscle aches, his diminishing memory, and his insomnia. Marshall observed that neither the orthopedic surgeon nor any of his colleagues ever asked him about his medications.

The neurologist saw him three days later. According to Marshall, the neurologist scanned through his recent history of having a mild heart attack, having stents placed into his heart, and taking several medications. After an examination, the neurologist considered the possibility that drugs might be a cause for his problems but wanted to be sure a stroke was not the culprit for his mental dysfunction. For these concerns Marshall received an MRI scan of his brain and had some separate specialized blood tests performed. When all these test results were reported as normal, the neurologist confessed that he was unsure what was wrong with Marshall.

Apparently, the neurologist was about to refer Marshall to an orthopedic surgeon for his leg complaints when he noticed in his own notes that his patient had already visited this doctor three days before. The neurologist asked Marshall to wait another week or two to see if his symptoms improved. If not, he wanted him to return for another visit. Meanwhile, the neurologist asked Marshall to continue his same medicines because they were good for his heart, and referred him back to the cardiologist. The cardiologist did not change Marshall's medications

By now Marshall expressed to me that he felt as if he were on a doctor merry-go-round.

By the time he returned to Sidney, Marshall thought he was getting worse every day. He telephoned the doctors in Billings, and it seemed that none of the doctors wanted to change his medicines for fear of hurting him somehow. Marshall didn't care. He just knew he felt awful and just wanted to be better.

The first thing I usually did when I saw patients like Marshall was to suggest to the patient that they stop all their medicines abruptly, if it could be done safely. In Marshall's case, I suggested he stop the medicines that made him sleepy and lowered his cholesterol because these were not needed urgently. I suggested he take half of the drug that slowed his heart rate. Finally, I suggested that he continue taking the two medicines to thin his blood, aspirin and a drug called Plavix, because they were part of a drug protocol to prevent clots in his new stents and were to be taken together for at least eight weeks. [30, 31]

Since Marshall and his wife had access to a computer, I gave them some references to refer out regarding the use of his medications in people his age and requested that he take some of those references with him when he went to see his cardiologist again.

Since I was asked only for my opinion, I made sure Marshall knew the decisions regarding his drugs and his body were his alone. However, I guaranteed him he would not die by following my suggestions. Furthermore, I asked that he confirm my suggestions with his other doctors for safety.

Marshall was asked to start a diary and enter how he felt that day, and he was to make a note in the diary every day at the same time. If he got worse, I wanted to know immediately; if he was somewhat better, he could tell me that too. Either way, Marshall was to return to my office in just a few days with his diary.

I knew the medication to lower his cholesterol, named Lipitor, was one of a class of medicines called statins. [32, 33, 34] These medications are notorious for having considerable adverse side effects in the elderly, most notably muscle aches, mental dysfunction, and insomnia. Why his doctors did not acknowledge these well-documented adverse side effects to the drug was puzzling to me. Additionally, this class of drugs is associated with a laundry list of other problems especially in the elderly patient. Fortunately, most of the problems resolve after the statin drug is stopped, but sometimes the muscle aches and pains will persist for a long time.

The medication to slow his heart rate was called atenolol, a beta-blocker class heart medication. [35] These medications in the elderly patient frequently cause fatigue, malaise, mental dysfunction, and sleep disorders. The dose of this drug was halved because I knew that stopping it abruptly had the potential of triggering another heart attack.

Since Marshall was already experiencing mental sluggishness, the sleep medication only would make this problem worse, so it was stopped.

I presented Marshall my reasoning for having him stop these medications, I wrote the reasons down on a piece of paper so he would not forget them and asked him to bring back my piece of paper with his diary when he returned. That way I would remember exactly what I had advised him to do.

Marshall did not call the next day, but the following day he called to tell me it felt as if a cloud was lifting from his head. His thinking was much better, but unfortunately his muscle pains persisted.

A few days later, Marshall called to tell me that he had researched his medications on the Internet. He exclaimed, "Those damn things are dangerous. I'm over seventy years old; I don't think I'll take them anymore. I'm going to tell everyone at cardiac rehab too."

By the end of several more weeks, Marshall was markedly better and, except for some residual muscle pains, he felt as if he were almost back to normal. His performance in his cardiac rehab sessions was improved, and he was sleeping like a baby without pills.

I informed Marshall that I had sent my notes about his improvement to his cardiologist, which he thought was a good idea.

About ten weeks after his heart attack, Marshall returned to my clinic after visiting with his cardiologist and his neurologist to discuss the conversations that he had with them. He related to me that after he presented the doctors with his list of problems, the articles about the serious side effects of the drugs they had prescribed for him, and his diary, he left their offices with only a prescribed healthy diet, an exercise program, and instructions to take a single aspirin tablet a day. [36]

EMERGENCY

You got to be careful if you don't know where you're going,
because you might not get there.

Yogi Berra

The Gunslinger

In 1979 with oil field activity in full swing, this Friday evening in our emergency room was absolute chaos. I had been busy caring for a variety of maladies for four or five hours. Now I was at the nursing desk completing my medical records. Our emergency room had four triage beds surrounding the nursing station: two beds were designated for patients with major medical problems and cardiac disease, and two beds were designated for minor trauma and miscellaneous problems. Down a short hallway from our main treatment rooms were a major trauma area, an orthopedic area, and a private room for performing gynecologic examinations.

Behind me in the cardiac cubicle was a gentleman having chest pain. I had confirmed that he had suffered a small heart attack, and he was waiting for a transfer to our cardiac intensive care unit.

Next to him was a teenager having an acute asthma attack. The nurse and I had been working with her for almost an hour to break her asthma spell, and it appeared the youngster was finally out of danger.

Down the hall in the orthopedic room was a young man waiting for his broken arm to be straightened. He had been riding a motorcycle, tried to jump a barbwire fence, and missed. While hitting a wood fence post at a great speed he sustained fractures of both bones in his left lower arm. Our anesthetist was attending him while he was preparing to take our young patient to the operating room for a reduction of his fractures.

In one of the other beds sat a middle-aged woman who frequented the emergency room with severe headaches. This woman had been evaluated in multiple headache clinics around the country trying to determine the cause. Doctors at the Mayo Clinic, the Diamond Headache Clinic, the Cleveland Clinic, and the headache clinic at the Johns Hopkins University had evaluated her. She did not have a diagnosis, but many physicians had prescribed multiple medicines which she took simultaneously to relieve her headache pain. Today her medications were not effective, and she was back in the emergency room requesting another morphine injection.

As I was completing my medical records and evaluating the laboratory reports I had received for my other patients, a young woman brought in a screaming, uncontrollable child with discomfort somewhere. I quickly ascertained the child was not acutely ill. The nursing aide in the emergency room escorted the young woman and her child to the minor illness evaluation bed. After a few minutes the child continued to scream even louder, throwing his body into gyrations suggesting to me that he was having nothing more than an attention-getting temper tantrum.

I heard a man's voice bellowing from the entryway to the emergency room call out, "Bobby, is that you?" Upon hearing the man's voice, the youngster stopped crying immediately.

I looked out into the emergency room doorway and saw an ominous appearing silhouette of a man backlit by the hallway lights. After he walked a few steps forward, I could see a tall, wild-eyed, middle-aged man standing in the doorway of the emergency room. He was wearing a dirty, torn long-sleeved shirt with the sleeves partially rolled up. His left forearm had what looked like a skull and crossbones tattoo. He wore dirty Levi jeans that were too big for him. On his left hip a large knife in a sheath extended down his leg halfway to his knee. I thought it looked like a Bowie knife. On his right hip a long-barreled revolver sheathed in a holster reached almost to his knee. A Buntline special, I thought, the kind of revolver supposedly used by Wyatt Earp. The holster was attached to an ammunition belt full of bullets that was slung around his waist.

Before I knew it, the man came up to the nurses' station, pounded his fist on the desk, glared menacingly into my eyes, and shouted, "Is that you making my boy cry? Huh?"

I calmly replied that I had not yet examined the youngster and told the man the screaming young boy had just come into the emergency room with his mother.

The man then exclaimed at me in a malicious tone, "If you hurt my boy, I'll kill ya! You got it?" He then looked toward the child and the woman and shouted, "Bobby boy, are these folks hurting you any?"

The boy did not say a word. We all could see that the man petrified the little boy.

The woman looked at this guy and said, "Honey, can't you see these folks are trying to help our son? Would you just come over here and be quiet."

The man complied by walking slowly toward the examination area next to his son and wife where he stood watching over me as I examined his five-year-old son. I could find nothing wrong with the boy except that he appeared to be a spoiled brat, had a congested nose with a bit of clear mucous, and had mild fluid congestion behind one of his eardrums.

I suggested to the mother that her child's problem required no antibiotics. In my opinion, her son appeared to have nothing more than a mild upper respiratory infection, a common cold if you will, and his problems should resolve within a week or so without any further treatment. By this time, the child was quiet, relaxed and not even whimpering.

However, it took some persuading for the father to believe his son required no antibiotics or further treatment. I handed the mother our standard handout instruction sheet for mild upper respiratory infections while the nurse encouraged the mom to call the hospital or to bring her child back if his condition worsened.

As the family was leaving, the father pointed his finger at me and proclaimed, "If my son's not better in a couple days, I'll be back." He then grabbed his wife's arm and led his family out of the hospital.

This man scared all the patients in the emergency area and me. I wondered what illegal drug he had been taking and what we would have done if he had become as menacing as he appeared.

I looked at the other patients in the emergency room. The woman with a headache had heard nothing after she received a morphine injection. The man with a heart attack was bewildered by the commotion but seemed no worse for wear. The teenager with asthma was frightened and having more respiratory trouble. We were able to relieve her symptoms promptly with more medication. The anesthetist and the boy with a fractured arm had already departed to the operating room.

This experience opened the eyes of all of us working that evening, and the incident was reviewed with the hospital administrator the next morning. By the next afternoon a sign was posted adjacent the hospital door stating the emergency room doors would be locked every night after 9 p.m. Beginning the next day, the hospital hired professional security staff to be available and visible in the hospital twenty-four hours a day and seven days a week.

When the oil boom sputtered and abruptly stopped in the early 1980s, the number of patients entering our emergency room on drugs declined dramatically. When the number of emergency room visits plummeted, the full-time security staff was discontinued after having been in force for almost two years. Hotline buttons with silent alarms to report unruly or dangerous patients were installed in the emergency room and at the reception desk that connected directly to the local Law Enforcement Center.

Sometime after this episode I read in the local paper that the same man in our emergency room had been arrested for trafficking drugs to our junior high school students and for felony assault. Soon thereafter he received a prison sentence.

Many times I have recalled this man's visit to our emergency room and thought how lucky we had been that night.

Elephants and Dragons

The first morning of my rotation in the emergency room as an intern included a basic orientation and a viewing of the general layout of the facility. Coming into the emergency room complex from the hospital revealed a wide-open area split in the middle by a large nursing station. To the left of the door was a large open area with four examination tables. Each of these areas was squared off with privacy drapes that extended from just below the nine-feet-high ceiling to just above the ground. To the right of the nursing station were two large rooms: one was for major trauma patients; the other was for acute cardiac patients and procedures. The nurse giving me the tour said I may get to be involved with something that occurred in the trauma room, but most assuredly I would not be allowed to go into the cardiac events room. She went on to say the Sacred Heart Medical Center was trying to develop a world-class cardiac surgery center and that acute cardiac patients would be attended by no less than the cardiologist on call and one or two heart surgeons as well as a nurse anesthetist who worked with the cardiac surgery team.

I asked the nurse why a physician anesthesiologist did not come to assess the patients rather than the nurse anesthetists. In her opinion, the cardiac surgeons wanted absolute control in the operating room, and in her view another doctor giving anesthesia just complicated the politics during the surgeries. Whatever the reasons, only nurse anesthetists were allowed to help with heart surgeries in this hospital.

We continued our tour by visiting the doctors' office area, otherwise known as the sleeping room, for the employed, full-time emergency room physicians. The two physicians I would be working with were Dr. Philip Little and Dr. Anthony Macintosh. I had the opportunity to visit briefly with the latter during my tour. He informed me that Dr. Little would start his shift about noon that day.

The emergency room nurse took me around to explain where things were located and offered that most of the time there would be a nurse available to get whatever I needed. However, just in case something was needed in a hurry, all interns were shown where to find materials and supplies that might be used during emergency situations including medications, instruments, resuscitation equipment, suturing materials, and casting supplies, etc.

When my orientation concluded after an hour or so, the nurse suggested I grab an early lunch so that I would be ready to start my shift at noon with Dr. Little. Following her recommendations, I made my way to the cafeteria, which was located three floors down in the hospital basement. Just before noon, I walked back upstairs to the emergency room to meet with Dr. Little.

As I entered the emergency room I noticed the drapes were drawn around all four of the examination areas. I saw nurses walking in and out of two of the rooms, and I could hear a man's voice, which I assumed was Dr. Little's, coming from behind the third set of curtains. From behind the first curtain, which was closest to me, I could hear a male voice moaning and groaning.

A nurse who appeared to be in charge of the emergency room at the moment and a person whom I had not met before came up to me and asked me if I was Dr. Ashcraft. (I thought this was polite since all the interns had prominent name badges on their white coats.) After I had confirmed my identity, the nurse called out and said, "Dr. Little, Dr. Ashcraft is here now."

I heard a man's voice say, "Good, I'm a bit busy sewing up this laceration. Have him see the gentleman in bed number one." The nurse consented and escorted me to the entrance of examination bay number one.

Behind the curtain I met a foul-smelling middle-aged man who reeked of alcohol, wore ragged, extraordinarily dirty clothes, appeared disheveled, and was curled up on his side in a fetal position. I carried with me a clipboard that held the man's emergency room record. I looked at the name of the patient on the medical record sheet and asked the man to tell me his name so I reconfirm that I was examining the correct patient. The man mumbled his name, and indeed it matched the emergency room record sheet.

I introduced myself and then asked him how I might be able to help.

The patient said he just didn't feel good and complained of hurting all over. The remainder of my history taking effort revealed very little because the man had difficulty remembering just about everything. He was not sure where he lived or of his birthday. He proclaimed to me, however, that he did drink booze once in a while just to stay healthy.

Since I did not get much useful information with my history

taking, I decided to perform a physical examination. I hoped I would be able to find something that would help me determine and resolve his dilemma. Since the nurse had already recorded the man's blood pressure, pulse, and respiratory rate, I did not have to obtain this data. On examining the man's eyes I noticed his conjunctiva were bloodshot and slightly yellow, and his pupils were dilated. The man's ears were covered with dirt, and it was apparent he had not bathed for some time. His mouth had few teeth with large dental cavities with severe gum disease.

My patient had already removed his clothes at the request of the nurse and had donned a hospital gown. I explained to him that I was going to listen to his heart and lungs.

He mumbled something in response which I understood as a consent.

After warming the head of my stethoscope in the palm of my hand, I placed it on the man's chest. (The tubing on the stethoscope is only about a foot long. Therefore, to listen to heart and lung sounds correctly the examiner must get close to his patient.) As I leaned forward toward his chest to begin my examination, the man threw his arms around me and pulled my face directly in front of his. Not only did I find out that this man was very strong, but he had body odor and breath that would gag a goat.

The man cried out, "Help me! They're out to get me! Don't you see them? Keep them from me!"

Because of his squeezing me, I was barely able to mutter, "Keep you from what?"

"The blue elephants and the dragons. Don't you see them?"

About this time I yelled out to anyone who could hear me that I needed some help.

I could hear Dr. Little's voice call out, "Hey Jim, what animals is he seeing today?" before he laughed out loud. Dr. Little continued, "Don't worry, Dr. Ashcraft, he's not going to hurt you. As long as you are between him and the monsters, he will feel safe now that you are protecting him."

I grunted that I didn't think I was being very helpful to anybody at that moment.

Dr. Little countered by telling me that in just a few minutes he would complete a laceration repair on his patient and would be able to assist me. He asked me to hang on for a little bit longer. I informed him that with the man's vise grip around my head, I really had no choice but to hang around.

Dr. Little did ask one of the nurses to go behind my curtains and see what she could do. The nurse came in, described the situation to Dr. Little, and informed him that everything was fine so far. All the time I was having this man blow his horrendous breath into my face. I thought I was going to unload my lunch on his face, but somehow I managed to keep it where it belonged inside of me.

After what seemed an eternity, but was probably only a few minutes, Dr. Little arrived and said with a big smile, "Hello, Dr. Ashcraft. I'm Phil Little. May I render some assistance?"

Before I could say a word, Dr. Little informed me that he knew this patient well and the patient was having yet another episode of delirium from acute alcohol withdrawal (called delirium tremens or DTs). [37, 38, 39] After reassuring me that he would extricate me from the man's clutches in a few moments, Dr. Little left the room and returned soon thereafter with a plastic intravenous fluid bag filled with a yellow liquid connected to some clear tubing and a needle. Still sporting a big cheesy smile, the doctor asked me to hang on for just a few moments while he quieted down my aggressive alcoholic. Without any objections from my patient, who was still gripping me vigorously, Dr. Little continued to insert the needle into a vein in the man's arm. When the needle was secured, he released the valve on the IV tubing and allowed the yellow fluid to flow into the man's arm at a maximum rate.

Within perhaps one or two minutes the man stopped seeing wild animals attacking him, released me from his bear hug grip, and lay on his side to rest.

As I pulled myself away from the man, Dr. Little said, "Welcome to the Sacred Heart Emergency Room." He continued smiling and chuckled out loud. As I looked around the examination area I saw all the nurses smiling too.

Before I left the area, the nurses placed a few restraint straps around my patient so he would not fall off his bed and allowed him to go to sleep right there in the emergency room.

Dr. Little took me aside where we had a short discussion about the patient. He told me the man was a Viet Nam veteran, a diehard alcoholic, and a frequent flier to the emergency room for various reasons related to his alcohol abuse, depression, and homelessness. On this occasion our patient was having yet another episode of delirium tremens related to alcohol withdrawal. Dr. Little explained that the IV fluid contained multivitamins and alcohol. (Alcohol was readily available in the hospital for intravenous use since, at the time, it was used in obstetrics to stop premature labor.) Furthermore, he told me that all he accomplished with the intravenous fluid maneuver was to give the man some vitamins to keep his delirium from getting worse and to give him an acute alcohol fix so the hospital could get him out the door quickly. Knowing the man's history, Dr. Little knew our patient would return soon.

By now our emergency room was beginning to fill up with patients, so Dr. Little said, "Dr. Ashcraft, There's work to be done and patients to see. We will talk when we have some spare time."

It was my first day in the emergency room. The day started for me at 8 a.m. Dr. Little and I finally had time to discuss our patients for the day at midnight. After another hour of discussing cases, I was pooped and needed some rest. I was on duty in the emergency room again at 8 a.m.

Just Kill Me Now

During one of my evenings working in the emergency room as an intern in Spokane, Washington, a man staggered into the reception area. Displaying the slurred speech associated with someone who had been drinking far too much alcohol, he declared that he was there to be killed. The man demanded that the receptionist get him to see a doctor who could kill him right now.

The receptionist really did not have to summon any of the physicians on staff because the man's voice was so loud and obnoxious that everyone in the emergency area, and probably the parking lot, could hear him. Both Dr. Macintosh and I were attending other patients behind the drape-lined cubicles when I heard Dr. Macintosh say out loud, "Oh my gosh, he's back." Immediately, he called for a nurse to find the man an examination area pronto.

I could hear people scurrying about in the emergency room as nursing personnel escorted this inebriated man to an examination cubicle. I overheard a nurse tell the man that the doctor could not see him until she was allowed to take his vital signs.

Despite his display of lewd, obnoxious, and abusive comments, the man was no match for the hardened, persistent ER charge nurse who succeeded in obtaining his blood pressure, pulse, and temperature. She then questioned him about when he last had a bath.

His reply with a slurred voice was, "It's none of your business." He then insisted that the nurse bring in the doctor to kill him because he was not going home again from the hospital unless he was in a coffin.

Dr. Macintosh and I finished with our patients at about the same time and met each other near the nursing station while we were completing the emergency room records for our last patients. Dr. Macintosh looked to me, pointed his head toward the cubicle with our obnoxious patient, and said, "Jim, he's all yours." He then gave me a great big grin.

Having grown up with an abusive alcoholic father, I am the first to admit that I have little patience with drunken individuals. I took a deep breath, gathered myself mentally and walked over to the examination cubicle. I pulled back the privacy curtains and slowly stepped into the examination area. The man looked at me and with a slurred voice asked me if I was the doctor who was going to kill him tonight.

Instead of answering him, I started to ask my own questions. To my question of how much he had been drinking, he proudly exclaimed, "One hell of a lot."

I asked him what he had been drinking.

The man struggled to sit up straight and with a slurred voice proudly reported to me that he had consumed a gallon of Ripple wine during the afternoon. He continued to say that he had tried to kill himself just before he came into the emergency room by consuming a bottle of Aqua Velva aftershave, a bottle of Listerine antiseptic mouthwash, some old, dried up, canned dog food, a mostly used bar of Ivory soap, and an old, dried up, moldy piece of cake he found on the ground beneath the Monroe Street Bridge. The man said none of these things killed him as planned, so he figured he just would come to the emergency room and have a doctor do it the right way.

Without examining the man, I thought I should start by vacating the contents of his stomach. In those days we used a product called syrup of ipecac to induce vomiting. At the time, almost every home had a bottle of ipecac syrup in an emergency kit to give to children or animals after they had consumed something that might have been hazardous.

I asked the man to wait while I walked out to the nursing area to get a supply of ipecac for him. I knew with certainty that I was not going to kill him.

I met with Dr. Macintosh, gave him the man's story, and advised him that I was going to administer some ipecac. He informed me that the man was a regular in the emergency room. The doctor also noted the patient had never asked to be killed. Dr. Macintosh smiled, patted me on the shoulder, and again wished me luck.

I took a small bottle of ipecac into the examination area where my patient was fading in and out of consciousness because of his alcohol consumption. When I aroused him, he asked if it was his time to be killed. I told him I wasn't going to kill him, but I had some medicine to give him to get rid of all the stuff he had been drinking and eating. I showed him the ipecac bottle.

The man looked at the bottle, and then looked at me with a blank stare, and yelled, "You're not going to get that pink grinch into me again. I want morphine! I want to die right here on the spot." The man then proclaimed that he was not going to move from his spot until I killed him and again demanded a large dose of morphine to put him out of his misery.

I returned to the nursing station where Dr. Macintosh, the nurse, and I had another discussion and decided that we should see the patient together. As we walked in to see the man, he pointed at Dr. Macintosh and said, "Hey man, I know you. Are you the one that's going to kill me? Did you bring the morphine? Did you know this other guy over there, pointing at me, tried to give me some more of that pink grinch crap?"

Dr. Macintosh affirmed to the patient that he had indeed seen him before in the emergency room many times and asked the man why he wanted to be killed.

Becoming impatient and more demanding, the patient expressed to us in specific and graphic terms what he thought of all our relatives and us and if we did not give him some morphine to die immediately, he was going to raise holy hell in the hospital.

I thought to myself this man was already raising a substantial commotion, and everyone within the confines of the emergency room, and perhaps the parking lot, could hear what he was saying.

Dr. Macintosh said to the man, "Okay, you win. I will give you some morphine. I promise you that if you do not die within ten minutes after I give you the morphine, I will give you another dose. Is that satisfactory?"

The man nodded favorably to Dr. Macintosh's comments and pronounced loudly that the doctor was a good man. The patient then reiterated his readiness to meet his Maker.

Dr. Macintosh and I walked over to the nurses' station to discuss what he had just promised the patient. Before I could say anything, Dr. Macintosh asked me if I'd ever heard of apomorphine.[40, 41] I admitted to him that I had not.

My mentor continued to tell me that apomorphine was a distant derivative of morphine with absolutely no analgesic properties whatsoever. However, it would make people vomit profusely. He said the local veterinarians commonly used the drug to make small animals vomit after they had ingested something toxic. He thought apomorphine would be a good solution for our dilemma.

Dr. Macintosh said, "This man wants morphine. We will give him morphine." He went to the drug cabinet and pulled out two bottles of apomorphine. One bottle contained medication that could be swallowed; the other bottle contained medication to be injected.

As we reentered the examination area, the man with his slurred speech shouted out, "Did you bring the morphine?"

Dr. Macintosh asked the man how he would like his morphine, in his mouth or in his butt. Then he showed our patient the two bottles of chemical. However, the doctor was sly enough to cover up part of the label with his fingers so that our drunken patient could see only the word morphine. The man looked closely at both bottles and insisted that he be given a morphine shot into his butt because he didn't want to risk not getting enough.

Dr. Macintosh reassured our patient that he would be right back. He then left the examining area but soon returned with several syringes filled full with apomorphine. He reaffirmed with the man that he wanted to receive the medication in his butt.

Our drunken patient yelled at us, "Quit talking and kill me right now."

Dr. Macintosh injected the syringe full of the medication into the man's buttock and again promised the patient that if he were not dead in fifteen minutes another dose of morphine would be given.

Our patient nodded in agreement and quipped that he hoped we gave him enough the first time. Again, he uttered that he was ready to meet his Maker. He thanked us and lay down on the examination table thinking he was just going to fall sleep and die.

Dr. Macintosh left the examination area but asked me to stay behind to watch our patient. Approximately two minutes later my patient looked at me and yelled out, "What the hell?" He just stared at me. He wanted to know if I was sure we had given him morphine.

I assured the man that he had been given morphine. Holding the bottle as Dr. Macintosh had done, I had him stare at the bottle again to reaffirm that the label said morphine on it.

As he was looking at the label on the bottle, the man started to wretch and vomit vigorously. I now realized my real purpose for being with the patient was to hold an emesis basin underneath our patient's face so he would not mess up the entire emergency room. Only the patient and I got covered with vomit.

When approximately fifteen minutes had passed, Dr. Macintosh returned to the examination area with another syringe filled with medication. Finding our patient still alive and with a sheepish grin, he asked the drunken patient if he was ready for his second dose of morphine just as the man was being overwhelmed with another wave of wrenching and vomiting.

When our patient stopped heaving, he shouted quite dejectedly, “Damn it anyhow. I can't even die with morphine.” He yelled out plainly that another dose was not going to be helpful and muttered dejectedly, “I guess I am just too damn tough to die even with morphine.” The man struggled to get up, stumbled as he barely made his way to the reception desk, said goodbye to the receptionist, and staggered out the door.

The entire emergency room staff had big smiles on their faces as our patient found his way out of the building, definitely not dead.

Dr. Macintosh looked at me and said quietly, "Don't worry, he'll be back."

Juan Juice

Between 1975 and 1981 eastern Montana and western North Dakota experienced its second oil boom in twenty years. Workers from all over the country came to our area in search of fortune and good-paying jobs. Not everyone came looking for jobs, however. Just like any other time in our country when there was a boomtown, a good number of inhabitants came to profit from the workers and their families.

Our emergency room saw patients with overdoses of drugs that were entirely foreign to our community. During medical training I had witnessed and cared for many patients experiencing the effects from a variety of drug overdoses. Nonetheless, in our rural community in eastern Montana, the majority of the overdoses were still from alcohol.

One Friday evening during the summer I was called to the hospital to care for a Mexican man the ambulance crew was transporting to the hospital. Because the patient was combative and barely controllable, the nurse wanted me to be in the emergency room when the ambulance arrived. Promptly I climbed into my Dodge pickup and drove the four miles into town from our country home.

When I arrived, the nurse informed me the ambulance was only a few minutes out of town. She said the ambulance personnel reported their patient was pretty much destroying the inside of the ambulance. The EMTs were trying to control him but were having only marginal success. They were driving the ambulance at the utmost speed allowed.

As the ambulance pulled into the garage located next to the emergency room, I could hear screaming and shouting coming from inside. The screaming and shouting was mostly in broken English but occasionally was interjected with short bits of Spanish. While quickly opening the rear doors of the ambulance to extricate the belligerent patient, one of the EMTs looked at me and said, "Doc, good luck with this one." as he displayed the bruises and abrasions on his face and arms he has sustained trying to control the man.

The Mexican man was obviously hallucinating and could not give us his name nor did he know where he was. However, he described distorted animals and people surrounding him. Terrified that he was going to die, the man was fighting off his demons by wildly swinging his arms and legs. In an effort to prevent any more hospital personnel from being injured, we held the man down with a full set of leather restraints, which included bands on his arms and his legs with a heavy strap across his chest. All of these were secured to the hospital gurney.

The ER nurse reported that the man's blood pressure was sky high, his pulse was racing, his pupils were dilated, and his mouth was terribly dry. I had the lab personnel draw some blood samples from which, hopefully, we could determine what this man had ingested.

As the emergency room personnel were trying to restrain this man, he described sounds that were making his ears burst, but there were no sounds. He described flashing lights and strange colors swirling around him, but there were no lights or colors that we could see.

After approximately fifteen minutes of wild and crazy activity, even with full restraints in place, the man became very placid. He started to smile and began to describe wonderful smells and beautiful colors in our emergency room. He must have told every female in the emergency room that they were the most beautiful pictures he had ever seen. He talked about now being able to see everything clearly and saying that he now understood the meaning of life.

Our patient had this quiet interlude for about half an hour before he reverted to his previous behavior of agitation, disorientation, and profound fear of being killed. He was terrified and was begging us to save him.

I knew our patient required close observation in the hospital. Yet, because of his disruptive behavior, I elected to keep him in the emergency room until I was assured that he would not be a danger to any more members of our hospital staff. We babysat this man in our emergency room for another two or three hours before he came down from his chemical high.

I thought the man's behavior to be reminiscent of patients I had seen in medical school who had taken LSD, the effects of which could last for many hours unless the person had been a perpetual user of the substance. In those cases, the trips from LSD could be considerably shorter. I hoped for the shorter version. [42, 43]

When I transferred the man to the hospital medical floor I hoped his hallucinations and his wild behavior had lessened, but I was wrong. For another twelve hours the man's behavior oscillated between being terrified and fearful to being calm, collected, and content. We maintained his full restraints the entire time. Fortunately, we had extra nursing personnel that day and were able to have one of our nurses monitor the man at his bedside continuously.

The laboratory technician informed me that she could not give me any help in determining what chemicals my patient had ingested. She could tell me, however, that my patient was entirely healthy from a biochemical standpoint. Although I thought this information was interesting, it wasn't terribly helpful in trying to determine how best to take care of my patient.

Even though I thought my patient probably had consumed some LSD, I could not confirm it. Also, I knew patients like this frequently took multiple drugs at the same time including marijuana, PCP, amphetamines, and others. Additionally, alcohol was usually involved.

The man seemed coherent and free of his drug ingestion about two days later. It was at this time that I questioned him about what he had consumed. The man informed me that he lived in Eagle Pass, Texas, and had come to our eastern Montana valley to find work. Unfortunately, he did not find as much work as he had hoped for which provided him with plenty of downtime. One day he and a friend decided to take some drugs just for kicks.

Finally, after what seemed hours of interrogation, my patient admitted that he had been using LSD off and on for some time. He revealed to me that LSD did not give him trips that lasted as long as they used to. In addition, he confessed to drinking one hell of a lot of alcohol but denied using any other illicit drugs. He blamed his friend for encouraging him to use a little bit of Juan Juice to boost the LSD effect.

To this, I asked him about Juan Juice.

In his Mexican dialect my patient explained to me that Juan Juice was totally safe and that I could buy it in the local grocery store.

I still did not know what he was talking about and again asked him to tell me exactly what Juan Juice was. The man stared at me with wide-open eyes and said, "Hey man, have you never heard of Juan Valdez?"

I agreed with the man that I had heard of Juan Valdez, the Colombian farmer in commercials for Folgers coffee.

My patient then exclaimed, "Man, now you've got it."

I answered that I still didn't think I had it and assured him that I really had no idea what he was talking about. I knew this man had not consumed enough Folgers coffee to make him act as goofy as he did. I asked him to tell me how Folgers coffee made him act so crazy.

My patient then explained how his friend convinced him he could increase the effects of the LSD by injecting some Juan Juice, i.e. Folgers coffee, into his veins. He went on to describe how he and his friend boiled some Folgers coffee over a campfire until there was just a thick goop remaining in the bottom of the can. His friend then added a little bit of beer to the can and mixed it up with the goop in the bottom. He then pulled some of the material up into a syringe and connected it to a needle. After my patient had placed a rubber band around his forearm to increase the size of his veins, his friend injected some of the material into a vein in his arm. This stuff was called Juan Juice.

I was amazed that someone would inject himself with coffee boiled to a slurry in a rusty can over a campfire without any pretense of being clean, much less being sterile, and not expect some serious things to happen.

I asked if he had any concerns about what he was doing by injecting this stuff into his body.

His only response was given with a big smile, "Hey man, Juan Valdez, he gave me quite a ride."

My patient left the hospital a short time later and was not seen again. Afterward, I informed the medical staff, the hospital staff, and the local law enforcement personnel that we now had LSD and Juan Juice being used in the Lower Yellowstone Valley.

Missing Tools

The 1974 World's Fair was held in Spokane, Washington, at the same time that I was completing my internship at the Sacred Heart Medical Center. Along with the volume of patients that the hospital usually experienced, there was a significant increase in the number of emergency room visits. My training time in the hospital's emergency room was continuously busy.

One Wednesday evening the emergency room physician, Dr. Anthony Macintosh, and I were experiencing standing room only business. We had nurses triaging the patients into groups: the slightly ill, the acutely ill, the acute trauma patients, and those patients with acute life-threatening problems. All of our examination tables and examination rooms were full. The waiting room was standing room only.

As I was busy suturing a laceration on a patient's face Dr. Macintosh called me from behind a curtain and said the ambulance had just arrived with a patient complaining of severe abdominal pain. The patient had been sent home from the hospital the day before after having had an abdominal surgery a week before. He said he could not get away from his patient and asked me to see the new admission.

I agreed to see the patient when I finished with my suturing, which I thought would take only a few more minutes. Dr. Macintosh replied that would be soon enough. Besides, he noted that the nurses first had to obtain the patient's vital signs and a preliminary history.

I completed my laceration repair and arranged for post-emergency room care for my patient with his usual physician, I then went to the cubicle where the ambulance personnel were waiting with the new patient.

The ambulance personnel told me that their patient was a middle-aged woman who had surgery performed by Dr. George Lucas at our hospital on Monday of the previous week. Apparently she complained of mild abdominal pain when she left the hospital two days before and reportedly had called Dr. Lucas that morning to tell him about her pain. She was reassured by her doctor and was asked to see him in the office the next morning. However, the woman reported to the ambulance personnel that her stomach pains intensified to the point where she could neither stand up nor walk, and she was having trouble urinating. The woman reported she had been hot and sweaty and unable to eat or drink because of severe nausea.

Entering the examination cubicle, I noticed a slightly obese middle-aged female who was pale, sweaty, and crying because of severe abdominal pain. I reviewed the records from the ambulance crew and the emergency room nurse outside the examination area before I went to the woman's bedside. After introducing myself, I asked about her pain and her other history. The information she presented to me was essentially the same that had given to the other medical personnel during this episode.

An examination of the woman was remarkable in that she had a recent surgical incision midline in her lower abdomen, and her abdomen was very tender to touch and rigid. Using my stethoscope I could not hear any noise in her abdomen suggesting a lack of intestinal activity. The woman's back was not tender. Her heart and lung examinations were unremarkable. After I completed the examination, I explained that I needed to discuss her case with my primary emergency room physician to decide what we would do next. The woman nodded that she understood.

Per hospital protocol, I discussed the case with Dr. Macintosh. Since the woman had called her surgeon earlier in the day and since the surgeon lived in town, I asked Dr. Macintosh if it was appropriate for me to call that physician before I continued with any further evaluation or testing.

Dr. Macintosh asked me the name of the surgeon. When I revealed to him the surgeon's name was George Lucas, Dr. Macintosh paused a few moments before advising me to complete my evaluation and to call Dr. Lucas after I had made a diagnosis.

After this discussion, I returned to relate this information to my patient who nodded that she understood. She just wanted some pain relief to feel better soon. I then completed my physical examination.

I requested the laboratory personnel to perform some blood tests and asked the nurses to arrange for the patient to have x-rays performed of her abdomen and chest. Within a few minutes the laboratory technicians had obtained blood samples, and the radiology technicians had escorted her on a gurney to the radiology department.

Perhaps fifteen minutes later I received a call from the radiology department. The technician requested that Dr. Macintosh and I come to the radiology department to view our patient's films because he saw something very interesting. I informed Dr. Macintosh of the phone conversation, and soon thereafter we went together to the department.

The technician had not yet removed our patient from the x-ray machine table thinking that we might want further studies taken before she returned to the emergency room.

The front-to-back image of the abdomen that Dr. Macintosh and I saw revealed two metal objects that had the appearance of metal surgical clamps. After I checked the patient's gown to make sure there were no instruments on top of her or behind her back, I asked the technician to take another exposure only sideways.

The technician said, "I just knew you were going to say that," and continued with obtaining a lateral view picture which revealed just what we surmised: the two metallic looking objects were indeed in the woman's pelvis. I looked at Dr. Macintosh and suggested it was time to call Dr. Lucas to see his patient.

Instead, Dr. Macintosh suggested that I call Dr. Edwards, the hospital's Chief of Surgery, to evaluate the patient first. Dr. Macintosh knew that Dr. Edwards was already in the hospital and could be in the ER quickly.

While the nursing personnel escorted our patient back to the emergency room, I paged Dr. Edwards to come to the emergency room and ask for Dr. Ashcraft.

When he arrived, Dr. Edwards seemed to be a very pleasant fellow presenting as a tall man in his fifties wearing a long white coat and looking professional. After short introductions, I presented my patient's case to him and then had him evaluate the x-rays that had just been taken. Dr. Edwards uttered, "I see," then asked to see the patient.

I followed Dr. Edwards into the examining cubicle to see the woman. After taking a very brief history, he recited some of the comments on the chart from the ambulance personnel and the nurses to the woman to verify her story. She affirmed the comments were correct. Afterward Dr. Edwards examined the patient and, without saying a word, he looked at me and said, "Let's talk outside please." The two of us exited to a quiet area and discussed the woman's situation. Dr. Macintosh joined us a few moments later.

Dr. Edwards told me that the woman's presentation was exactly as I had described. He agreed that she definitely had an acute surgical abdomen and needed an operation urgently to remove the surgical tools that had been left in her abdomen by Dr. Lucas.

I mentioned to Dr. Edwards that I would call Dr. Lucas and discuss his patient, but he intervened with a firm voice, "No, I will call George. We appear to have a problem." Dr. Edwards immediately went to the telephone and summoned Dr. Lucas to the emergency room.

Dr. Macintosh and I went back to care for other patients in the emergency room. However, we asked the emergency room nurse to notify us when Dr. Lucas came to see his patient.

A short time later, a stocky, overweight elderly man came walking rapidly into the emergency room. He had sweat on his forehead so I assumed that he had been moving briskly. The nurse directed him to me and said, "Dr. Ashcraft, this is Dr. Lucas."

After I presented my patient's situation to Dr. Lucas, he said he wanted to see the x-rays that I had taken. Subsequently Dr. Lucas and I, accompanied by Dr. Macintosh, went to the x-ray viewing area in the emergency room. When Dr. Lucas saw the two surgical clamps on the x-ray he glared at me and said, "Young man, is this a joke or what? There is no way those instruments are in my patient's abdomen." Dr. Macintosh intervened and said, "Yes George, the tools are in your patient's abdomen."

About this time, Dr. Edwards came into the x-ray viewing area and asked to be alone with Dr. Lucas.

After their conference, Dr. Edwards and Dr. Lucas returned to the emergency room, and Dr. Edwards invited me to accompany them to the patient's bedside. After a few introductions and some informal small talk, Dr. Lucas advised his patient that there appeared to be a dilemma related to her surgery, but he did not specify the dilemma. He told her that he had asked Dr. Edwards to assist him with another operation to correct the problem. The woman agreed and uttered to us she just wanted some relief from the pain in her abdomen. Dr. Lucas assured his patient that they would take her to surgery soon and make her feel better.

Afterward, Dr. Macintosh took me aside in a quiet area of the emergency room to inform me that this was not the first time Dr. Lucas had left something in a patient's abdomen. Since Dr. Lucas had been on the hospital's medical staff for a long time, the doctors were hoping that he would retire without hurting anybody else. Still, he continued to perform surgeries on a weekly basis. His usual surgical procedure was a hysterectomy (removal of a woman's uterus) with a suspension of the bladder, which was the surgery he had performed upon this woman. Dr. Edwards was asked to examine the woman to see firsthand Dr. Lucas' surgical complications. After this discussion, we went back to take care of still more patients in the emergency room.

As my emergency room shift was concluding near midnight, the charge nurse informed me that Dr. Edwards requested to see me in the doctor's lounge when I was done. So when my shift was completed, I went to visit him. Dr. Edwards was waiting patiently in the doctors' lounge eating a snack. He invited me to sit down, put my feet up, and take a break. First, he congratulated me on a job well done in evaluating the woman for which I thanked him. He then asked me to look at two surgical instruments lying on a nearby table that had been extracted from Dr. Lucas' patient. Fortunately, the patient did not appear to be infected. Dr. Edwards said he would assume the woman's post-surgical care and planned to keep her in the hospital for about a week. He invited me to follow the patient's progress as well. We talked for a short time about a few surgical issues, and then I went to bed.

When I went to see the woman in her hospital room a few days later, she said that she was feeling dramatically better. In particular, the severe pain in her abdomen was now gone, and she was able to eat and get up to walk without much difficulty. I asked how often the surgeons came to see her. She replied that Dr. Edwards usually visited with her in the morning and in the evening. She said Dr. Lucas had left her room just before I came in and explained to her how he had found a small problem with the way a couple of small blood vessels had been clamped. He apparently assured her that the problem was corrected and she should have no more trouble. The woman thought Dr. Lucas was, "Such a very nice man."

What the doctor didn't tell his patient was that the problem with the blood vessels being clamped was that he forgot to remove two clamps from inside her abdomen. She could have died from complications. I learned a short time later that the seventy-one-year-old Dr. Lucas was asked by the hospital's medical staff to retire. He did so immediately.

It's All Your Fault

Beginning in the early part of 1980 reports appeared in the American medical literature of young, previously healthy young men dying of cancers and infectious diseases that formerly had been seen only in the elderly. Before their deaths, these young men developed a severe body wasting disorder that was unknown. The only thing these patients had in common was that they were homosexual.

By 1982 an increasing number of reports emanated from medical centers in New York, Los Angeles, San Francisco, Atlanta, and Seattle with descriptions of an increasing number of similar cases with this wasting disease. In the original reports it appeared that the life expectancy of the patient after the disease process started was less than two years. Furthermore, the disease process now appeared to be, for the most part, confined to a certain group of individuals who were characterized in the media as being one of the "4 H Club": heroin users, homosexuals, hemophiliacs, Haitians (An unusually large contingent of these victims was from Haiti, especially in New York).

Although its cause was undetermined, by the end of 1982 the disease itself was given the acronym AIDS (acquired immune deficiency syndrome). From the information supplied by the media and the medical establishment, it was difficult for anyone to distinguish what was true, what was false, and what was made up about AIDS. The way the disease was transmitted remained obscure, which allowed the media and special-interest groups to speculate wildly.

In April 1984 simultaneous announcements were made in France and in the United States that researchers had determined the cause of AIDS to be a viral infection. The virus was given multiple names by different researchers but eventually was given the name HIV (human immunodeficiency virus). [45, 46, 47, 48]

Soon thereafter the United States government charged several companies in the pharmaceutical industry with developing a test for the virus. By March 1985 Abbott Pharmaceuticals developed the first commercially viable blood test for identifying the human body's antibodies to HIV. To ensure safer blood products, all the American blood processing companies promptly started using this product.

I had a discussion with one of the members of the Montana State Health Department in the winter of 1985 about AIDS. At the time he informed me that the number of AIDS cases in Montana was fewer than twenty and that none of these individuals had been infected in Montana. He informed me that, as far as he knew, all were individuals who had come home to die. During the conversation, this individual suggested to me that my chance of seeing an AIDS patient in eastern Montana was about as good as my house being hit by a meteor on the Fourth of July.

Despite reassurances from this health department employee, who supposedly knew the latest information about AIDS, and because I was receiving frequent requests from people locally and in nearby towns to talk with groups and schools about AIDS, I decided to go back to school. In the fall of 1985, I participated in a two-week mini fellowship on AIDS at the University of Washington Medical School in Seattle, Washington, where I attended many lectures about AIDS. Additionally, I observed patients and physicians in community HIV clinics for the indigent, I spent time with a gay physician whose entire practice was dedicated to middle class HIV patients (who, by the way, had the means to pay), and I observed the care of AIDS patients in special areas of the University hospitals. I garnered plenty of information to deliver to the individuals and groups I would address in the future.

About 8 o'clock one March evening in 1986 I was in the hospital because the dreadful wintry weather outside prevented my going home. I was reading in the doctor's lounge when I heard a page over the hospital intercom to report to the emergency room STAT. Instinctively, I dropped what I was doing and ran toward the emergency room. As I was coming down the corridor to the emergency area, I saw a pool of blood splattered on the floor inside the hospital entrance door and a trail of blood leading into the emergency room. Upon entering the emergency room, I saw a young man lying on a cot with several hospital personnel around him. He had blood on his shirt and his face, and I noticed another pool of blood on the floor from yet another episode of vomiting.

I asked the nurse's aide if she had been able to get a blood pressure and vital signs. She said the man's pulse was fast, his blood pressure was low, and she could feel his pulse barely. I knew that if this man was not yet in shock, he soon would be so I asked the emergency room nurse to call the lab technician to obtain blood for testing and to cross match some blood immediately while I grabbed a nearby IV supply tray so I could insert an intravenous catheter. As I was inserting the intravenous catheter into his arm, I tried to reassure the young man that he was going to be all right.

He responded by crying out, “What the hell do you know? It’s all your fault, you know. What do you doctors know anyway?”

I told him we needed to stabilize his blood pressure first and stop the bleeding. When we got his hemorrhaging controlled, I assured him that he would be fine. The young man cried out again, “I'm going to die, and you know it. So don't lie to me.”

I thought the young man to be hysterical, so I ignored his outbursts. When his vomiting of blood stopped a short time later, I thought it might have ceased because his blood pressure had dropped low enough so that the remaining blood had time to clot. I inserted a second intravenous line into his alternate arm and, after I saw that the IV fluid was flowing well, secured the line to his arm with tape.

His laboratory data suggested that he was severely anemic and would require a blood transfusion to replace his lost blood. Fortunately, his blood type was O positive, the most common type. I did not believe the man’s emergent situation would allow the lab tech the two hours needed to process the blood completely, so I had the lab tech deliver two units of O positive blood to the emergency room that had been typed only and not tested for antibodies. To do this, I was required to sign papers to waiver any liability for the hospital. I then started the blood transfusions in the emergency room.

Sometime later after his vital signs had stabilized and his bleeding had stopped, I had an opportunity to talk with my patient. When I asked him to tell me little bit about himself, he just started to laugh. I asked what was so funny about being in the hospital and throwing up blood. Looking away from me with his eyes rolled upward he replied, “If you only knew.” I assured him that I had plenty of time to talk, if he wished. The first thing he said to me was that he was going to die and that we were going to die with him. Again he stared at me and said, “It was all your fault.” He was mad that we had kept him alive.

I asked him to clarify what he was saying. He revealed to the emergency room nurse and me that he had AIDS and he was dying. The bloody vomit all over us was infected so we were going to die just as he was. He pronounced to us with a wry smile, “What about them apples?”

I knew that nothing was going to happen to us just because we had HIV infected blood on our clothes. I knew the AIDS virus was not transmitted that way, but I did not argue with him. I mentioned that he appeared to be very upset about something to which he angrily exclaimed, "Damn right! I'm twenty-four years old, and I'll be a dead man in six months!"

This declaration seemed to open up the floodgates for him to talk. He informed the nurse and me that he came from an ultra conservative small community in North Dakota and he was gay. Since he was the only son of four children, his parents not only expected him to take over the family farm, but also to get married and produce grandchildren. Instead of coming out about his homosexuality with his parents, he moved to San Francisco soon after finishing high school where he met his boyfriend who had died about six months before. Our patient was diagnosed with AIDS at the same time. Since then, he lost his job, became unable to pay his bills, accumulated a large medical debt, and finally was forced to tell his conservative parents in North Dakota what had happened to him.

Apparently, the young man's father demanded that he stay in California and die; his mother, however, pleaded with him to come home. He had decided to return home just a few days before. The young man ended up in our hospital because he ran out of food, his car was out of fuel, he had no money to rent a place to stay, and he started throwing up blood soon after he arrived in town. He wanted to know what I thought now.

I told him he was a sick young man who vomited a lot of blood, and we at the Sidney hospital would do our best to care for him.

The young man received about six units of blood and spent several days in our hospital to recuperate. An endoscopy revealed just superficial ulcers in his stomach, which I hoped would heal nicely with the appropriate treatment.

It was interesting to me that several of our nurses and doctors wanted nothing to do with this patient. I did not question them if they were refusing to see him because he was gay, because he had AIDS, or for some other reason. Fortunately, the remainder of our staff treated him like any other sick patient. He was the first AIDS patient many of them had seen.

While the young man was in the hospital, the local clergy collected donations which allowed him to refuel his car and buy food for the remainder of his journey back to his home in North Dakota.

After my patient was discharged, the doctors, nursing staff, and administrative staff of the hospital convened a conference to review and modify the hospital's guidelines and protocols to protect our personnel from infected bodily fluids. All the people involved with this case had HIV testing done immediately and six months later. All the results were negative.

Not long after this episode I had an opportunity to talk with the same individual at the state health department with whom I had talked before. I informed him, "The meteor did not hit my house on the Fourth of July, but I did see a patient with AIDS." His sarcastic response was, "Crap happens to the best of us."

Sometime near Christmas in 1986 I had a conversation with one of our local ministers. He wanted to know if I recalled a young man with AIDS who came to our hospital one wintry night some months before. I told the pastor that I recalled the episode quite well.

He informed me that through his church contacts he learned the young man made it to his home in North Dakota safely. He said the man was able to make amends with his family and died at the family farm in the summer.

In the time since this episode, information has evolved that proved the HIV virus first appeared in patients in Africa sometime between 1890 and 1930 and appeared to be a mutation from a similar virus that was prevalent in certain monkeys. By evaluating blood from people who had died from curious unknown causes, scientists have been able to identify the first cases of AIDS in Europe and the United States from the late 1950s and early 1960s. Africa had experienced an epidemic of patients dying with a fatal wasting disease from an unknown cause for perhaps thirty or more years before AIDS was identified elsewhere in the world.

When my patient's AIDS diagnosis was made in 1986, his life expectancy was less than two years because no treatment was available. In the subsequent two decades, diagnostic tools and treatments emerged for the HIV infection and its related disorders. AIDS was transformed from a death sentence into a chronic disease lasting twenty or more years if the patient could afford the treatment.

The cost of medications in the United States alone in 2010 was about $25,000 per person per year. The combined costs of care for an AIDS patient at the same time approached $60,000 per year, and most of this expense was paid through some form of government funding. [48, 49, 50]

A Routine Emergency

During the peak of the oil boom in Sidney, Montana, the hospital contracted with a physician group to provide full-time coverage for our emergency room. As a rule, the physicians this group supplied performed well. Unfortunately, a few of the doctors just were not made to work in emergency situations. One of these physicians was Brian Van Buren, M.D.

Since Dr. Van Buren had recently come out of the military where liability issues were of little concern, his new employers had impressed upon Dr. Van Buren that if a patient came into the emergency room and the patient thought he had an emergency, then the physician was to treat the patient as though he indeed had a real emergency.

Being military trained, Dr. Van Buren considered this to be an order to be obeyed and no deviation was allowed. If the patient said he needed a service, then it was his job to deliver that service, no matter what.

When the telephone rang I was in a deep sleep. At the other end of the phone I heard an excited voice yell out, "Dr. Ashcraft, Dr. Ashcraft. This is Van Buren in emergency room. It is double aught thirty-six and I have a . . ."

In my sleepy stupor, the first thing I heard was "double aught thirty-six." I thought only of thirty aught six (30.06), the rifle caliber, and quickly sat up on the side of my bed and asked, "How bad is the gunshot wound?"

The next thing I heard was, "Dr. Ashcraft, sir, It is double aught thirty-six. Excuse me, sir. It is thirty-six minutes after midnight Saturday morning, sir. I have an emergency for you."

I asked the doctor if there had been a gunshot accident.

He replied, "No sir."

After I took a deep breath, I asked Dr. Van Buren to tell me about his emergency.

Again, with a rapid cadence in his speech, he yelled into the phone, "Dr. Ashcraft, sir, I have a man who wants a vasectomy."

Still in a sleepy fog, I responded, "Van Buren, are YOU kidding me?"

He replied, "No sir, I am dead serious."

I explained to Dr. Van Buren that a vasectomy was not an emergency procedure, and I performed it in my office. Besides, preliminary counseling had to be done with the man and his spouse before the procedure.

After a few seconds Dr. Van Buren replied, "Hold on Dr. Ashcraft. I'll get back to you."

After perhaps another thirty-seconds or so, I heard Dr. Van Buren on the phone. He said, "Dr. Ashcraft, the man really wants to have a vasectomy done today. He says his insurance runs out Monday morning. That is less than forty-eight hours from now. You won't be paid."

I informed Dr. Van Buren that insurance companies usually did not pay for vasectomies anyway. Besides, I was not coming into the emergency room in the middle of the night for someone I had never seen to perform a vasectomy. Of course I wouldn't be paid because I wasn't going to do it. I told him it was a stupid idea.

Again, the doctor asked me to hold on for a minute.

When he returned, Dr. Van Buren continued, "I relayed your message to my patient. He said if that's the situation with his insurance, then he'll just go back down to the Mint Cafe with his friends and drink a few more beers.

I questioned the doctor if the man was drunk.

"Dr. Ashcraft, sir," he responded, "I am reasonably confident that the man appears to be intoxicated." There was a momentary pause before the doctor resumed. "By the way, Dr. Ashcraft, the patient and his friends just left the emergency department. Sorry to bother you. Have a good night sir." I heard a dial tone.

All I could think of was, "What a bonehead!"

I had no problem going back to sleep. The emergency was over.

A Surgical Emergency

The Veterans Administration Hospital (the V.A.) at the University of Oregon Medical School in Portland, Oregon, was constructed in the late 1920s. Like many government endeavors refurbishments and updates to the facility were done on a priority basis and when taxpayer funds became available. When I performed my medical school general surgery rotation at the V.A. in the summer of 1973, the buildings were over forty-five years old and desperately in need of upgrading. Unfortunately, money at the time was diverted into high tech medicine, and the areas that received the upgrades were in the cardiac intensive care units, the cardiac radiology departments, and the cardiac surgery suites. These areas had and promoted the most modern equipment. The remainder of the furnishings in the buildings of the V.A. complex were, for the most part, the originals from 1928.

The entire general surgery suite area was a collection of rooms of various sizes where surgical cases were scheduled depending upon the surgery being performed and the surgeon. In the summer afternoons some of these rooms became quite uncomfortable because there was no air conditioning. Only the heart and brain surgeons had air conditioning in their surgical suites.

One day the first-year surgery intern and I were scheduled to assist a local private surgeon named Phillip Scheidecker. Dr. Scheidecker performed surgery at the V.A. for free once every two weeks so he could help the veterans and teach doctors-in-training at the same time. We had three surgeries scheduled on this day with the first operation scheduled to start around 8 a.m. Dr. Scheidecker figured we would complete all the cases by noon and then he would allow time for some one-on-one teaching with the students before he left for the day.

The first operation was supposed to be a simple abdominal wall hernia repair in an obese man. Unfortunately, as Dr. Scheidecker tried to open the hernia, he found a large, rock-hard mass that was definitely a cancer. Instead of taking about an hour to complete a simple hernia repair, this procedure turned into a major cancer operation which lasted almost four hours. The entire team needed a break before we could start the second operation.

The second operation was another hernia repair. Thank goodness the surgery went as planned and was completed within an hour. It was now after two o'clock in the afternoon, and the operating room was becoming stifling. The only way to get some ventilation into the room was to open a row of windows that were located high above about ten or more feet up the outside wall and to open the surgical suite doors. This was a very hot summer day; the sun was shining directly into the windows.

While the team was preparing the room for the next surgery, one of the nurses took a long pole with a hook affixed to one end to release the latches on the windows high above and push them open. I noticed some air movement but not enough to counteract the heat that was streaming in.

The third case was the removal of an inflamed gallbladder in a quite elderly veteran. Just as Dr. Scheidecker opened the patient's abdomen, a large bug passed directly over the wound about a foot or so above the patient. Dr. Scheidecker asked, "How did that bee get in here?" One of the nurses replied that the bug was just a very large fly and not a bee. Dr. Scheidecker asked the surgical supervisor to dispose of the creature before it contaminated the patient's wound.

With this instruction, the nurse retrieved a fly swatter and attempted to bring down the pesky little insect. With such a high ceiling in the operating room, the fly easily flew up out of harm's way whenever the nurse tried to swat it. After a short time, the fly deserved the attention of two nurses trying in vain to knock it out of the air.

As our surgical team worked diligently to remove our patient's gallbladder before the next fly attack, we heard a swoosh sound. A second swoosh got us to look away from the operating table to see a third nurse trying to knock the fly out of the air with sprays from a canister containing tincture of benzoin, a sticky substance used to stick surgical drapes together. The spray traveled quite a distance but all that I could see happening was that the nurse was putting sticky red-brown spots high up on the walls; she never came close to the bug as it kept escaping high into the vaulted ceiling.

Dr. Scheidecker called out, "Listen up people, what we have here is a surgical emergency." He then said, "Doctor Ashcraft, (He called everyone in training doctor. I liked that.) Since you are the tallest one in the room, would you please try to get rid of that doggone creature before it contaminates this man's wound?" I immediately stepped away from the operating table and grabbed another fly swatter.

I was standing behind the anesthesiologist at the head of the table when the fly landed on his anesthesia apparatus. I swatted and missed, and again the insect flew to the safe haven of the high ceiling.

In just a few seconds, the fly started to circle over the surgical table again. I just happened to be behind Dr. Scheidecker when the fly landed on the back of his surgical cap. Without thinking, I made a powerful swat at the insect and hit the doctor squarely in the head. I heard him say, "Ugh" as his head wobbled from the impact of my blow.

"Well, did you get it?" he asked. I told him I was sorry that I hit him. He, however, was more concerned with the fate of the oversized fly than his head. I told the doctor that I was not sure and asked him to allow me time to search for the fly's remains.

One of the nurses exhorted that she was sure that I got it.

After a cursory viewing of the impact zone on Dr. Scheidecker's head, I found the remains of our elusive enemy smashed into his surgical cap. He had one of the nurses apply a new surgical cap over his old one so that none of the beast would ever get into the wound. After his new cap was in place, Dr. Scheidecker raised one arm and proclaimed, "A significant victory over pestilence!" He declared the need for a celebration in the hot operating room and ordered orange juice for everyone.

By now I did not need to reenter the operation since the gallbladder was out and the intern was closing the wound. Afterward, Dr. Scheidecker came up to me and thanked me for my stealth in killing the fly. He assured me that when he came to the V.A the next time, he and I would remove a gallbladder together, and I would be the primary surgeon. Quite a fine reward for squashing a fly I thought.

The next day, I saw flypaper hanging from the high ceiling in front of all the open windows.

ALL ABOUT KIDS

"Do Not believe in Miracles. Rely on them."

anonymous

Betsy Flights

In May 1974 the Watergate scandal in Washington was coming to fruition with the beginning of the impeachment proceedings of President Richard Nixon. The Vietnam War was coming to closure and finally would be over in the spring of 1975. Literally hundreds of thousands of American military personnel were returning home.

At the same time, there was a proliferation of activity in medicine. Hospitals were competing to see who could become the first or the best in their area to provide advanced services areas such as cardiac surgery, intensive cardiac care, hematology, advanced laboratory techniques, and orthopedic replacement surgeries. This competition occurred as hospitals and physicians tried to gain greater market shares of their local and regional populations.

Sacred Heart Medical Center in Spokane, Washington, where I interned between 1974 and 1975 was no different. Its competition was the Spokane Deaconess Hospital located only a few blocks away. As in many cities there was tremendous competition and rivalry between the Catholic-run hospitals (Sacred Heart) and the Protestant-run hospitals (Spokane Deaconess).

While I was on my pediatrics rotation at Sacred Heart Hospital, my fellow intern on pediatrics and I were asked one day if one of us wanted to go out to pick up a sick baby in a nearby town. The trip would involve taking a ride in a helicopter. My colleague had no interest, so I jumped at the chance. I was instructed to be ready to leave from the helicopter pad on the roof of the hospital in thirty minutes. (I didn't even know there was a helicopter pad.) After completing a few incidental tasks, I grabbed my doctor bag and headed to the roof of the hospital.

A nurse from the pediatric intensive care unit met me at the exit door to the helicopter landing pad. She brought with her an incubator that had been modified so it could be fastened to the floor of the helicopter. She quickly showed me how to connect the incubator to special attachments inside the helicopter on the floor and then left me standing there with my incubator awaiting the arrival of the transport helicopter. I was excited. I thought I was going to take a ride in a new shiny white helicopter.

After I had been waiting about five minutes, a faded, camouflage-green colored, military Huey helicopter from nearby

Fairchild Air Force Base came in for a landing. As it approached the designated landing area near me, two airmen leaned out the side doors to guide the pilot onto the pad. The helicopter appeared just like the ones that we saw in the newsreels of the Vietnam War transporting troops into battle and carrying casualties away from the battlefields. After the helicopter landed, one of the airmen came over to me and grabbed my arm to escort me into the cabin of the helicopter. He placed headphones on my head and buckled me into my seat securely. The other airman grabbed the incubator and put it next to me in the cabin and together we secured the incubator to the floor of a helicopter. I looked forward and saw a pilot and a copilot.

The copilot turned around through the opening in the cockpit and spoke into his microphone, "Doctor, welcome to Betsy One."

The copilot asked me where I was going. After I mentioned the name of the town where the hospital was located, he said, "That's a good thing doctor, because that's where we're going too." He gave me instructions on the operation of the headphones followed by introductions for himself, the pilot, and the two wingmen. The wingmen then closed the doors to the Huey helicopter, and the captain called out, "Is all secure?" When the wingmen affirmed both doors were secured, the pilot said, "Gentlemen, let's retrieve a sick baby." The helicopter then lifted off without incident, and we were on our way.

En route to the hospital about seventy-five miles away, I talked with the two wingmen about their military experiences in the Air Force. The entire team and the helicopter had returned from Vietnam just a few weeks before. Apparently, according to one of the airmen, they needed to maintain their skills, and the hospital needed a transport vehicle for sick babies. Thus the idea of the Betsy flight was conceived. (One meaning for Betsy is humanitarian.) I was on this team's inaugural Betsy flight for Sacred Heart Hospital.

As we were nearing the hospital, I heard the pilot say over the intercom, "We have our destination in sight gentlemen." He asked the other three airmen where he should land because apparently there was no designated landing area. Remember, this was the maiden voyage.

The copilot pointed out a parking lot or an empty field perhaps a block or less away from the hospital that was wide open and without any visible obstruction. One of the wingmen pointed out a parking lot near the hospital emergency door that was much closer.

The pilot said, "Well, let's just go down and take a look see," then steered the helicopter in a circular pattern around the potential landing sites near the hospital complex. The pilot, noting that telephone wires surrounded the area next to the hospital, requested the copilot to estimate the width of the landing area adjacent to the hospital.

After the copilot gave him his best guesstimate of the size of the parking area, the pilot said, "We can make it. No problem." Quickly turning the helicopter around so that it was soon above the landing area, the pilot gave an order for the wingmen to prepare the doors for landing. At that point the two airmen opened the helicopter doors and stretched out supporting themselves by one arm and a foot support that was inside the helicopter. Each of the wingmen then called out to the pilot the distances of clearance for the helicopter blades. In what seemed to be a routine maneuver, the pilot guided the helicopter down expertly without incident into the small landing area surrounded by telephone wires.

While the pilot turned off the helicopter and went through his checklist for shutting down the machine, the wingmen assisted the infant incubator and me out of the helicopter. As I pushed the incubator toward the hospital, one of the airmen from the cockpit shouted, "Doc, good luck. We will be here when you're ready to go home."

Two nurses met me at the hospital door and escorted me promptly to their nursery. Since no doctor was around to give me a history, the nurses directed me to their sick, fourteen-month-old baby girl who was moribund. She was floppy, pale, and mottled. I looked at the chart to find that the child had been diagnosed with meningitis several days before, and, to my surprise, she had not been fed and intravenous antibiotics had not been given. Fortunately, some of the baby's spinal fluid had been obtained and cultured as evidenced by the laboratory results.

About this time, I received a telephone call from the local doctor who screamed at me that it was about time I got there. According to the elder physician, the baby was damn sick and was going to die. However, the doctor did not want the baby to die in his hospital on his watch.

I asked the doctor if he had tried to insert an IV into the child.

The elderly physician informed me that they didn't do that

kind of fancy stuff at his little hospital. That's why he called the big boys from Spokane to take care of this sick child. The doctor rudely demanded for me to "get that sick kid out of my hospital!" He hung up the phone before I could respond.

After I examined the little girl, I called the pediatrician working in the intensive care unit at Sacred Heart Hospital. I gave him the child's history, the laboratory results, the results of my examination, and the comments made by the elderly physician.

The pediatrician at Sacred Heart advised me that the elderly physician was probably right about the baby. It was obvious to him the doctor had made some errors in the management of the child's meningitis and was looking for a way to save face in his community. The pediatrician asked me to load up the baby and just head home.

I asked the pediatrician if he wanted me to start an intravenous line and start giving the baby some intravenous fluids and antibiotics before we left.

He suggested that it was best under the circumstances to leave quickly. He thought I could start the IVs when I arrived back at the home base.

With assistance from the local nurses, we bundled the infant into the incubator, collected all the records, and went out to the helicopter. After the airmen helped getting the incubator and me secured inside the cabin of the helicopter, Betsy One took off toward the Sacred Heart Hospital in Spokane.

Once back at Sacred Heart, the incubator and I were assisted out by the airmen. Before my departure, the pilot said, "Doc, I hope you enjoyed the flight. Perhaps we will see you again another day."

With the assistance of the nurses waiting on the helipad, the infant incubator with its seriously ill infant passenger aboard was transported to the pediatric floor and then into the intensive care unit. There the pediatrician with whom I had consulted evaluated the child. He agreed with my assessment. The pediatrician allowed me to insert two intravenous catheters into the child's legs: one was for fluids and nutrition, and the other was for antibiotics.

My job was done for my first Betsy flight; I returned to the general pediatrics floor to resume my duties.

As we anticipated, the baby was profoundly ill and died several days later from bacterial meningitis despite some heroic efforts by our pediatric intensive care staff.

I was fortunate enough to fly on eight Betsy flights during my intern year. I helped care for sick babies that were born in hospitals in the small Washington communities of Ritzville, Ellensburg, Othello, Wenatchee, Chelan, and Mary's Lake. I also flew on a nighttime Betsy flight that used only radar guidance through the mountains and valleys on our way to Sandpoint, Idaho. I have to say that while the airmen were having a grand time flying in the dark, I was scared.

As the years passed and hospitals developed their own medical specialty programs, many added their own helicopter and airplane transport programs to pick up sick and injured patients. Later on, many hospitals considered these programs too costly and abandoned them. Sacred Heart Hospital eventually stopped its relationship with the military transports and started its own air transport program.

As for me, I had the opportunity to be just a small part of a pioneering humanitarian effort to retrieve and save sick infants called Betsy flights.

Bless His Heart

The nurse's note on the chart hanging outside the examination room door read, "Major little boy problem." My nurse had a way of piquing my interest before I entered an examination room.

A pregnant young mother was sitting in the room with her three-year-old boy Lawrence. She brought her little boy into my office this particular morning because he had something wrong with his "male thing." The mother related that her little boy had cried most of the night because his peewee hurt. This morning when she looked at her little boy's penis, she saw that it was covered with a foul smelling gray gunk. The mom and her husband knew that something was not quite right with their little boy, and she brought Lawrence promptly to the clinic instead of the hospital emergency room.

Lawrence was whimpering. When I asked if I could help him, Lawrence just pointed to the front of his underwear and cried, "It hurts."

I asked the little boy if I could take a look inside his pants.

He nodded and then pushed his underwear down to his ankles so I could see his genital area. I noticed immediately that Lawrence's penis was not circumcised. His penis was red, swollen, and hot to touch with pus coming out from under a foreskin that extended well beyond the end of the penis. This condition is called an infected phimosis.

I informed the mother that her son's problem was caused by an infection in the oils and other material that collected underneath his uncircumcised foreskin. The current condition would worsen with time because the intense swelling of the tissue could decrease the circulation to the penis. I also informed the mother that the only way to have a definitive treatment for this problem was to circumcise Lawrence.

The mother was against circumcision, at least she thought so until she saw the amount of pain her little boy was having. She wanted to know if the condition could be corrected with antibiotics and more cleaning.

I told the mom that cleaning under the swollen foreskin would require pushing the foreskin back toward the base of the penis. This action, along with the tremendous tissue swelling, would do nothing more than to have the retracted skin act as a tourniquet on the already inflamed organ. This only would make the situation worse, in my view. I suggested that she allow me to circumcise her child that day and correct the problem.

The mother responded by asking me to give her a few minutes to think about what I had said and to make a telephone call to her husband to discuss the situation.

I escorted the mom into my office to use my private phone.

In the meantime, I asked the mother if it would be okay if I brought my nurses into the exam room to see her child. I explained to her that her son's condition was not seen very often, and I always was looking for ways to educate my staff. She nodded yes.

While the mother was telephoning her husband, I summoned my nurse practitioner and my nurse to the examination room. When the mother returned from making her phone call, I showed my two employees Lawrence's problem. I explained that Lawrence's problem was caused by his penis being uncircumcised, having a stricture in the foreskin, and having an infection in the material that collected under the foreskin. I asked the two women to examine the inflamed, swollen organ carefully.

Roxanne, my nurse practitioner who had recently moved to Sidney from Tennessee, squatted down next to Lawrence, examined his penis without touching it, and said with her southern accent, “Bless his leettle haart.”

For some reason, her comment was very amusing to me and, without thinking, I said, “I don't know where you were trained, Roxanne, but where I'm from, that thing is not called a little heart.” Roxanne looked at me, thought about what she had just said, and exclaimed, “Oh Mercy me. I am so sorry.” She blushed and just smiled. I smiled and chuckled too.

Lawrence's mother said she and her husband agreed to have their little boy circumcised, and she wanted to know when the procedure could be done.

I told her that I would check with the operating room to see if I could do it over the lunch break that day. She agreed and noted that having the procedure done quickly would be good for everybody, especially Lawrence.

Once I explained my little patient's predicament to the surgical team, they assured me that there would be no problem in performing the procedure over the lunch break. As long as Lawrence had not eaten anything for one hour, the anesthetist was comfortable with giving him an anesthetic.

I was certain that at least an hour had passed since Lawrence had eaten anything. Therefore, I scheduled the surgery. I informed the mother that I would be able to perform the circumcision promptly and asked my nurse to arrange for the little boy to be admitted to the hospital for the procedure.

I performed the circumcision procedure without incident; Lawrence had to remain in the hospital just a few hours for observation before he went home. I arranged with the mom to bring her son to my office for a reevaluation of his penis in two weeks.

Lawrence and his mother returned to my office as I had requested. He was now a much happier little boy. His penis had healed nicely and now appeared normal. I asked Lawrence if his peewee hurt anymore, and he emphatically said No! I asked the mother if she had witnessed any difficulties with Lawrence after his surgery, and she replied no.

Before they left my office, I asked Lawrence and his mother to wait a few moments while I retrieved my nurse practitioner because I wanted her look at my handiwork.

Roxanne ventured into the examination room, greeted Lawrence, and asked the little boy if she could look at his peewee again. Laurence nodded and pulled down his underwear.

Roxanne squatted down to the floor, looked at the little boy's normal appearing, circumcised penis and said, "Bless his leettle haart." She looked up at me and smiled.

Lawrence and his mother left my office on their way to the Dairy Queen. I gave them a prescription for a free lunch on me as I did often.

For many years my nurse practitioner and I had a running joke that whenever I would show her something different or unusual, one of us would say, "Bless his leettle haart."

A Bit of Luck

On a late spring day in the early 1990s a young mother went into labor near her due date and had an unremarkable birth of a viable, healthy eight-pound baby girl. The parents named their baby Tonya.

Per the hospital routine, the newborn girl was taken to our nursery for her preliminary observation, stabilization, and care. The mother was returned to her hospital room. All seemed to be good and routine.

The baby had been in the newborn nursery several hours when I received a call from the nursery nurse who told me that the baby had been out to see her mother to breastfeed. After she returned to the nursery, the nursing aide was feeding Tonya when all of a sudden the baby started to make grunting noises and appeared to be having difficulty breathing. The nurse also revealed to me that the baby had a low-grade fever.

I knew that newborns should not be febrile. I also knew that the baby should not have respiratory troubles unless something was drastically wrong. A thousand things raced through my mind as I ran to the hospital nursery from my office which was located about a hundred yards away.

Upon my arrival in the nursery, I noticed the female infant had grunting respirations, pale mottled skin, and diminished muscle tone. These signs all suggested to me that the infant was having an acute respiratory event of some sort. I surmised that the newborn might have aspirated while feeding or was infected since these were the most common reasons for acute respiratory distress in a newborn. The presence of a fever suggested that the baby might be septic.

After my evaluation, I inserted two catheters into the blood vessels of the baby's umbilical cord. From these catheters I obtained blood for testing to check for any infection and to determine the degree of respiratory impairment. Additionally, the catheters would be used to give the baby fluids, to administer antibiotics, and to obtain more blood for laboratory testing as needed. I knew that with small babies one must expect the worst and treat for the worst as quickly as feasible. Any significant time delay could be the difference between a good outcome and a poor one. The infant was started on oxygen given through a mask, and potent antibiotics intended to kill the most common bacteria found in these circumstances were started intravenously.

X-rays were performed, which revealed a good placement of my umbilical catheters and no evidence for any acute problems in the lungs. Unfortunately, I knew that x-rays often did not reveal changes of a lung infection for many hours or days after the baby was ill.

Unfortunately, by the time the x-ray films returned, the baby suffered a respiratory arrest and required ventilation with a bag and mask. After a short time, I had to insert a catheter into the baby's airway and connect her to a mechanical ventilation machine.

After I had performed these maneuvers and the baby appeared to be stabilized, I spoke with the neonatologist in Bismarck, North Dakota. Together we discussed the option of an air transport for the child. Unfortunately, because of some technical problems, the air flight team out of Bismarck was unavailable for an unknown time. Since I was unable to transport the baby, I advised the neonatologist that I was comfortable managing the child on the ventilator for a short time since I had done it multiple times before. I also was aware that I did not have the experienced nursing staff to provide continuous care for the baby for too long. The doctor assured me that he would contact me when the air flight service was available again. I reciprocated by telling the doctor I would keep him informed of my patient's condition.

By now, the entire obstetrics wing was abuzz with activity regarding our sick newborn baby. I made my way to the mother's room to notify her that her baby, who seemed healthy only a few hours earlier, was now struggling too survive, and I had no answers for her. I could explain to the parents only what I had done, whom I had consulted, and what we all planned to do in our efforts to make their baby well.

After another eight hours, baby Tonya appeared to be breathing much better, and the ventilator was discontinued. She started to spit up some discolored mucus which made me think that she may indeed have aspirated something while she was feeding, and I knew that the x-ray findings of a possible pneumonia from aspirating might not be visible for several days. I remained concerned that the baby might have an abnormality of the esophagus that would provide a direct connection between the food tube and the air tubes in the lungs. Therefore, I arranged for the radiologist to perform a special swallow x-ray the next day.

The next morning the radiologist performed the special

swallow procedure and found no abnormalities. To me, this was very good news, and one of my concerns about this baby's illness was eliminated.

After twenty-fours hours Tonya's respiratory status was much improved. Not only was she breathing by herself off the ventilator but also she was requiring a minimal amount of additional oxygen to keep her blood oxygen levels at a normal value. About this time, the laboratory bacteriologist informed me that the blood cultures I had obtained the day before grew a large amount of a bacterium called group B streptococcus. [51, 52, 53]

Again I consulted the neonatologist in Bismarck, North Dakota. I discussed with him my baby's progress, the laboratory and radiology results, and questioned whether a transfer to the newborn intensive care unit was still necessary.

The neonatologist informed me the air transport was now unavailable because of bad weather. Furthermore, he did not think the baby needed to be transferred to his facility and suggested that the baby be given intravenous antibiotics for ten more days.

Additionally, the neonatologist gave me a teaching session regarding group B streptococcus in newborns by explaining that the mortality rate for newborns that became sick with group B streptococcus within the first day was about fifty-five percent. Apparently death was not caused by the bacteria itself but rather by a toxin that the bacteria produced.

Group B streptococcus is a normal inhabitant of the human body with approximately forty percent of women being colonized with this bacterium in their genital tract at some time during a pregnancy. It is unknown why only a few newborns are predisposed to becoming infected by this bacterium during the labor process.

Tonya's parents could see that their baby was improving; I kept them and nurses updated frequently.

Tonya remained in the hospital on intravenous antibiotics for another ten days. Her mother was allowed to breast-feed her, and this natural process went without any incidents. When the course of antibiotics was completed, the umbilical catheters were removed, and the baby was allowed to go home with her parents.

After Tonya, I had the opportunity to treat twelve more babies with group B streptococcus over the next few years. I had not seen any cases before baby Tonya, and after obstetric care guidelines were developed to screen and care for moms with group B streptococcus a few years later, I saw no more cases.[54, 55] Two of the babies with group B streptococcus that I did treat died, but thankfully the numbers were not close to the published fifty-five percent mortality rate.

I had the good fortune of watching Tonya grow and develop until she was about seven years old. Her family moved away from Sidney when her father decided to return to college at an out-of-state institution. When the family left the community, Tonya had developed normally, was smart, and was doing well in school.

I heard about the family about ten years later when an acquaintance told me they had moved back to a small community in Montana. I learned Tonya had developed normally, was intelligent, and was near the top of her high school class. Like any other teenager in a small school, she was active in many activities.

About a year later, my wife Kay and I had the honor of presenting an academic scholarship to Tonya when she graduated from high school.

Tonya wrote me a wonderful letter stating why she desired to attend college to become a lawyer and help disadvantaged people. Eighteen years earlier I was not sure Tonya would survive the day. Now she was a bright young woman going off to college with a promising future.

I thought what a fine reward for me for having a bit of luck on that eventful day so many years before.

The Things Kids Say

A young woman came to my clinic to see me along with her three-year-old daughter for a routine matter. While the woman and I were talking in the examination room, the daughter sat on the floor and kept herself busy with a coloring book. All of a sudden the youngster exclaimed, "Doctor, Do you have a hairy bum like my daddy?"

The mom and I were both startled by this outburst. Giggling, the mother replied, "Aurora, be nice."

Before I could say a word, the little girl continued, "Did you know my mommy has hair on her twinkie? My daddy says someday I will have hair on my twinkie. I'll have big boobies like my mommy too.

The mother exclaimed, "Aurora Jean, hush right now!"

Unfazed, the little girl sat on the floor and continued to color pictures.

The mom's face was flushed.

I didn't say a word.

A young pregnant patient who was about seven months' gestation was in my clinic for a routine prenatal visit. On this occasion, she brought along her two-year-old son because she wanted him to hear the baby's heart beat.

After my patient was on the examination table, I asked the little boy if he wanted to hear the baby's heart beat. He nodded, and I pulled a chair alongside the examination table and lifted the youngster onto the chair so he could be closer to his mom's abdomen.

"Why is Mommy's belly so big?" the little boy asked.

I told him that his mom had a baby inside. I then used my ultrasound unit to listen to the baby's heart tones. I held the little boy's hand on his mom's abdomen so he could feel the baby move.

The little boy then asked, "Why is Mommy's butt so big?"

"Daniel," the mother immediately responded, "enough with the questions!"

I didn't say a word.

The child remained silent for the remainder of the examination.

A mother and her three-year-old daughter journeyed to my clinic from their ranch outside town for the child's yearly well-child examination.

I was answering the mother's questions about her child when the little girl asked, "Doctor Jimmie, Did you know my mommy loves my daddy a whole lot?" The little girl stretched her arms wide open to show me just how much.

I replied that I was sure they loved each other very much.

She replied, "You want to know how I know?"

I told her I would love to know how she knew that her mommy loved her daddy a whole lot.

"When my daddy comes in from the pig barn all dirty and smelly," she shouted, "my mommy tells him he is the most handsomest man in her world. Then she smushes on his dirty face with her mouth. Oh gross!"

The little girl let out a great laugh.

The mom just smiled.

I smiled and continued with my evaluation. Afterward, I told the little girl she had made my day and gave her two coupons for ice cream cones at the local Dairy Queen.

Kay and I were sitting at a table in a mall cafeteria in Orlando, Florida, when a little girl, whom I guessed to be three to four years old, came walking by accompanied by a middle-aged couple I guessed to be in their early sixties. The little girl was wearing a full-length red dress and shiny new shoes. I guessed they had just come from the Walt Disney store.

I greeted the little girl by saying, "Hello, pretty little person."

The little girl stopped in her tracks and stared at me. She put her hands on her hips, put on a face of indignation, and exclaimed, "I am not pretty. I am **beautiful**!" After a short pause, she shouted, "I'm a **princess.**" Again shouting, she added, "I'm **really smart** too. I'm a **really smart** and **beautiful Princess."**

She looked up at the man at her side, fluttered her eyelashes, and said softly with an impish smile, "Aren't I grandpa?"

I smiled and said, "Yes you are, My Lady." I bowed my head in respect.

After a short pause, I looked at the little girl and stated, "You're an independent young lady too."

She stared at me and exclaimed, "I am not. I'm with my grandpa." She then grabbed his hand.

The grandparents just laughed, smiled, and walked away.

The Daredevil

On a warm spring Saturday afternoon I was called to the emergency room by a nurse who informed me that there had been a farm accident and a four-year-old boy had been injured severely. The youngster was being brought to the hospital by his parents. The nurse asked me to be in the emergency room when they arrived.

Not knowing what kind of trauma the child had sustained, I asked the nurse to inspect all the pediatric resuscitation equipment in the emergency room before the patient arrived. I got into my pickup truck and drove the four miles from my home in the country to the hospital.

The youngster and his parents arrived just a minute or so before me. I could hear the youngster screaming as I walked down the corridor to the emergency room, so I surmised the patient was not in any acute distress from a heart and lung standpoint.

When I entered the emergency room, there was a throng of people making a considerable amount of noise and a great deal of uncontrolled commotion. As I made my way to the bed where the child had been placed, I noticed a male child who appeared to be in no acute cardiovascular or respiratory distress. Readily I could see multiple superficial abrasions on his face and arms. Despite the child screaming uncontrollably complaining of pain in his leg, the nurse assured me that his vital signs were good.

While the nursing personnel removed the little boy's clothing with scissors, I cornered the parents to ask them what happened. The family indeed did live on a farm, but the event that injured their child was not actually a farm accident. The mother told me that they had recently bought three-wheeled all-terrain vehicles (ATVs) for the entire family. They even got a small vehicle for their four-year-old son. The father had shown their little boy how to drive the ATV and had watched him practice riding out in the field. Consequently, the parents were assured that their son could control the vehicle.

"These parents thought their little boy was strong enough to control a fifty horsepower off-road vehicle?" I thought to myself. "What were they thinking?"

The father explained that their son, unbeknownst to them, built a ramp next to a collateral irrigation ditch so that he could jump over the ditch with his new ATV. Apparently a family hero was the famous daredevil Evel Knievel from Butte, Montana. The father noted that his son only had to jump about eight feet to span the ditch and be safe. After viewing the crash site, the father concluded that his son's vehicle left the ramp going too slowly. Soon after the ATV left the ramp, the front wheel dipped down, and the vehicle impaled itself into the sidewall of the irrigation ditch. His son subsequently was thrown from the vehicle another ten to fifteen feet into a cornfield injuring his left leg. Upon arriving at the scene of the accident, the dad noticed that his son's left leg was crooked beneath his pants. He then picked him up, laid him in the seat of his pickup, told the family members he was going to the hospital, and then raced into town.

By now, the little boy's clothes were off, and I was able to evaluate him more thoroughly. Indeed, his left leg was crooked over the thighbone. Furthermore, I observed many more bruises and abrasions on the youngster's torso, back, and right leg. I placed a splint on the little boy's left leg to stabilize the fracture and sent him to the radiology department for x-rays.

The pictures revealed a clean, angulated fracture in the middle portion of the left femur. I reviewed the x-rays with the parents and advised them that I would have to put their child to sleep to set the fracture. I explained the process required to stabilize the fracture to the parents and obtained their consent to perform the procedure before I called the hospital's surgical team leader. At the suggestion of the anesthetist, I gave the little boy an injection of medication to alleviate some of his pain.

Within a short time, the surgical team escorted the youngster to the operating room where he was given a general anesthetic. With the aid of two surgical technicians I was able to straighten the fracture and apply a double leg hip spica cast to stabilize it without much difficulty. A double leg hip spica cast means that a continuous plaster cylinder was applied from the belly button to the toes on the fractured leg and to just above the knee on the uninjured leg. A bit wooden bar was incorporated into the cast across both upper legs to provide support for the cast and to provide a handle to move the child. The boy was then moved to a hospital bed for observation.

Over the next couple of days, the youngster complained of minimal pain, and the cast did not need to be modified because of swollen tissues. Our physical therapist instructed the parents on how to care for the cast, carry the child with the cast, and how to manage caring for their son's bodily functions through the large opening that was made in the cast. The boy left the hospital after three days.

Leg radiographs repeated a few days later reconfirmed that the femur fracture was still in good alignment. Also at this time I was able to answer a list of questions the parents had for me. I explained to them that the healing time for their little boy's leg was unknown, but at his age, a femur fracture usually required about eight to twelve weeks. I told them that I would take x-rays of his leg in another week to verify its alignment and that any further treatments would be decided upon then. I gave the parents written instructions for the follow-up plans.

Fortunately, the femur fracture healed without incident in three months. During the healing process interval, I learned that this little boy was a bit of a hell raiser, and as his grandmother observed, "He was just like his father."

I removed the boy's cast at the three-month visit after his x-rays revealed a completely healed bone. I advised the parents that their son might require a week or so to get back up to full speed because his leg muscles would be weak after being immobilized for such a long time. I requested that they bring their son to my office in another two weeks for a final evaluation.

When the little boy literally ran into my exam room two weeks later, it appeared to me that he was definitely near full capacity regarding the use of his legs. I congratulated the little boy and his parents on a job well done.

The father related that since his son's three-wheeled ATV was severely damaged by the accident, he and his wife had decided it was too dangerous for their son to use it; so they didn't get the machine repaired. (All three-wheeled ATVs were banned in the United States in 1987 because of deaths and safety issues related to the vehicles' instability at higher speeds and with rollovers.)

Finally, these parents have come to their senses, I thought to myself. I expressed to them that, in my view, they had made a wise decision. The father displayed a big grin when he said they recently had ordered their little boy a little motorcycle for Christmas. I wished them good luck.

When the child and his parents left my office that day, I feared that I would see him again soon with a severe motorcycle induced injury. It never happened. As the years passed, the little boy developed into an accomplished motocross racer. His parents encouraged him every step the way, despite his injuries.

The Cattle Buyer

One early spring day I had the opportunity to visit with an eight-year-old girl who had accompanied her mother to the clinic. While my nurse assisted the little girl's mother with her medical needs for the day, the little girl showed me a picture of her holding two baby lambs. She proudly told me that these were her 4-H project lambs and that she would raise the animals during the summer and finally sell them at auction during the County Fair. The little girl invited me to see her lambs at the County Fair in the fall when they were full-grown. I told the little girl that I would be honored to visit her and her lambs at the fair.

In the latter part of July of that summer, I saw the little girl and her father one weekend while I was shopping in town. The little girl ran up to me, showed me a new photograph of her with a grown lamb, and reminded me of my promise to visit her and her lamb at the County Fair.

The little girl's father thought his daughter was bothering me and encouraged her to come with him. I assured the dad his daughter was not a bother. I told her that I remembered we had a date to meet at the County Fair. The little girl smiled and said, "Okay." She then took her father's hand, and they continued shopping.

The County Fair was held every year in early August. I always enjoyed walking through the animal barns and the agricultural exhibits. While my family and I were making our way through the 4-H animal exhibits, we met the little girl and her mother with her prized blue ribbon lamb. The girl was combing the lamb in preparation for the judging which was to be held that day.

The mother asked us if we had ever been to the 4-H auction. I said I had not. The mother invited my wife Kay and me to attend the 4-H auction that day to watch her daughter demonstrate her lamb before the buyers because she thought we would enjoy the event. She said, "Who knows, you might even buy a lamb." The mother informed us that the auction was always held at a certain time in the afternoon right after lunch. As we were making our way further down the animal exhibits, the little girl called out and said, "Hope to see you at the auction Doctor and Mrs. Doctor."

Kay and I really had no intention of going to an animal auction. However, while we were walking around the fairgrounds, we met Ann, one of the hospital nurses, and her husband Dan who farmed north of town. While we were discussing what we had seen and done at the fair that day, Kay mentioned our visit with the little girl and her mom in the 4-H barn.

Dan commented that a good share of the 4-H kids were probably my patients and thought it would be good for me to be seen at the 4-H auction. Besides, Dan thought we might even bid on an animal. Kay noted that she would not know what to do with the lamb. Dan assured us that pigs and steers were also for sale. He explained to us that many people went to the auction just to see the animals and to observe the youngsters' presentation skills. There never would be an obligation for us to buy anything. Again, Dan thought it would be a good idea for us to go to the auction just to see some of my patients outside of the office.

The four of us had lunch together at the baseball booth where we discussed among other things the 4-H auction. When the announcement for the 4-H auction came over the fairground loudspeakers, Kay and I accompanied Ann and Dan to the auction arena.

We arrived at the auction arena in plenty of time and even had time to go into the 4-H barn to look at the animals one last time before they went up for sale. The animals had the ribbons they had received during the earlier judging on display by their stalls. It was during this short walk through the animal barn that Dan convinced us that we should bid on one of the animals just to get our feet wet.

As the four of us settled onto the bleachers of the auction arena, Kay and I decided that we would buy one of the steers. However, I asked Dan to bid for us because I couldn't understand what the auctioneer was saying. Dan smiled and replied, "Not a problem," but he wanted to know how large a steer we wanted. We told him that we didn't have a clue. I personally knew nothing about buying steers and had no idea how much meat a steer would produce.

Dan asked, "Do you want to bid on the Grand Champion steer for publicity, a blue ribbon steer, or one that you're going to eat?" Certainly, I had no idea what he was talking about, and I asked him to explain the differences.

Dan explained that the blue ribbon steer was usually the biggest and the fattest in the lot. A local business usually bought this steer for publicity to show their support for the kids. Blue ribbon steers, as a rule, had more fat. The red ribbon steer had considerably less fat but, in his opinion, produced the best eating meat. Dan then pointed toward a group of men sitting in a specific section of the bleachers. He revealed to us that these individuals were cattle buyers and never bought the blue ribbon steers. Their jobs were to get the best meat for the best price. He suggested that if we didn't know what to do, we could wait until the buyers started bidding. We then would know when the steers that produced the best meat were coming up for bid.

As I recalled the old medical school adage, "See one, do one, teach one," I told Dan he still could bid for us this time. I figured that this was the one that I would see.

The auction started as Dan further explained to us how to evaluate the different steers as the 4-H kids paraded their animals around the arena. He showed us how to tell which steers were too fat and added that the red ribbon steers usually sold for considerably less money per pound than the blue ribbon steers.

Dan selected an animal for us and bid until he offered the winning amount. Afterward, he said, "Now, wasn't that easy? You are now the proud owner of a 4-H steer." Dan explained to us how and where we paid for the animal, where the animal would be taken for processing, and who we would contact when it was time to pick up our meat.

Kay and I met with the animal's owner, who happened to be one of my pediatric patients. After having our picture taken with the child, we presented a check to the child to close the transaction. Later on I would put the picture in my office collection of kid pics.

A few weeks later our meat processing was completed (all seven hundred pounds of it), and we invited Ann and Dan to our house for a barbecue with our 4-H beef. Dan said that he liked rib eye steaks best, so we had barbecued rib eyes for dinner that evening.

Kay and I found out that the amount of meat from a single 4-H steer easily met our family's beef needs for an entire year.

The next year at the county fair, Kay and I decided that we would buy another 4-H steer because the meat was superb and we had an opportunity to support another child. This time we selected a steer that belonged to one of the children who came to our clinic, and I bid on the steer at the auction while Ann and Dan watched me. Kay and I found that there was a certain amount of personal satisfaction that came with winning a 4-H auction and having your picture taken with the youngster who raised the animal. Besides, the picture always went into my kid pics gallery in my office and became a conversation piece.

Since we had a growing family and enjoyed the 4-H meat, we continued to buy 4-H steers at the county fair. Kay and I decided that the most important criterion for the animal was that it had to be raised by one of the children in my medical practice.

One year the price of beef was quite low. The blue ribbon steer that normally would bring up to one dollar fifty cents per pound sold for only ninety-five cents per pound. The subsequent steers were selling for only sixty to sixty-five cents per pound or less, and it seemed to me that the kids had put in an awful lot of work not to receive more compensation for their efforts. Overhearing our discussion, a rancher sitting next to me at this auction told me, "The kids have to learn the cattle business and sometimes prices are pretty darn bad, like now. Sometimes you can't give the darn critters away."

Kay and I had selected a steer to buy this year that was raised by one of my pediatric patients. The girl was one of a pair of twins I had delivered. The bidding started at fifty cents a pound. With the bidding hovering around fifty cents per pound and not progressing very fast, I bid seventy-five cents. The auctioneer called out, "Doc, it's yours."

The next animal for auction belonged to the other twin and again, the bidding started at a low price. Nobody would start the bidding on this steer. The auctioneer tried to encourage the people in the audience to support the kids. Kay nudged me with her elbow and whispered, "Why don't you bid just once to get things started?" I was hesitant but bid anyhow. I called out, "Sixty-five cents to get things started." The auctioneer called out, "Doc, you got another one."

I wondered to myself, "What are we going to do with two steers?" It seemed that I had put my foot in my mouth again. Kay and I were shocked and amused at our dilemma. What were we going to do with TWO steers? Together we decided that we could find places for the meat.

The butcher wanted to know how we wanted our meat cut, so we decided that the majority of it should be ground into hamburger. That way we could give the meat away to different groups for fundraising activities. After the two steers were processed, we had over fifteen hundred pounds of meat. Over the months that followed we were able to give significant amounts of hamburger to the Boy Scouts, the Girl Scouts, the hockey team, the high school booster club, and the 4-H kids to help them with their yearly fundraisers. Kay and I still had plenty of meat to feed our family for the rest of the year.

We continued to bid for and buy 4-H steers for many more years.

For The Kids

Kay and I were fortunate when we moved to Sidney, Montana. The community provided us with an excellent education system, a safe environment for our children to grow up, friendly people who taught us how to be good neighbors, and a place where I could practice medicine.

Many people had helped Kay and me in many ways along our journeys through high school, college, medical school, and beyond. After a short time in Sidney, we felt an obligation to begin returning the many favors that we had received over the years.

Periodically, my office staff, who knew everybody that came into our clinic, and I would sit down with our ledgers. They would tell me about the families with children who could not pay their outstanding balances and often we decided to eliminate the debts. The patients received a birthday or a holiday gift bill from the clinic with a zero balance.

We found that kids in the nearby counties were constantly having fundraisers for some worthy project. My clinic had an unwritten rule that if a youngster, not the parent, solicited a donation in person, a donation was given. My clinic donated to many causes over the years.

When Kay and I were asked to assist with a worthwhile community endeavor such as the local museum, the Boy Scouts, the Girl Scouts, 4-H clubs, the local hockey team, the local baseball association, and, of course, school sports and activities, we never refused.

One of the side effects of getting involved with kids in a small community is that you get asked to be involved in all sorts of ways. With our children participating in many activities, Kay became involved too. She served on the School Board and coached the successful freshman girls' volleyball team at 6 a.m. While our children were in school, she became the coach, the bus driver, the cheerleader, the snack food vendor, and the counselor for our kids and their teammates when they participated in extracurricular activities at home or on the road.

One day while we were eating ice cream cones at the local Dairy Queen restaurant, my son David, who was about ten years old at the time, asked me, "Dad, why are you and mom such do gooders?" I asked him what he meant by do gooder. He replied that it seemed to him that his mom and I did a lot more to help kids than the parents of some of his friends and classmates.

I informed David that his mom and I did not have parents who got involved with us very much when we were kids, and we were just doing what seemed like the right thing to do. I asked if our efforts bothered him. David replied, "Nope, I like it."

In the early 1990s, Kay and I decided to focus our charity efforts toward kids going to college. Like the scholarship I received many years before that allowed me to attend Eastern Montana College, we decided that our scholarships would be awarded without a formal application to qualified high school students chosen by us who wanted to attend college. It became our way of letting the kids know that people other than their immediate families appreciated their efforts through the years as they grew up.

Over the years, we have been gratified to receive notes from some recipients who revealed to us that they would not have been able to attend college without our help and that we made a big difference in their lives. To make things even better, most of the scholarship recipients were kids I helped bring into this world. Since we started giving scholarships, Kay and I have been fortunate to help about seven hundred high school graduates take advantage of higher education.

HELP ME

"A strong positive mental attitude will create more miracles than any wonder drug."

Patricia Neal

Let Me Die

I met Rachel and Vernon during a weekend in the hospital when I was taking calls for one of the other doctors in town. This couple was in their late sixties and had a ranch not far from town that had been in their mutual families for multiple generations dating back to the late1800s.

On this occasion Vernon was in the hospital with respiratory difficulties. Vernon had been a cigarette chain-smoker since his teenage years and had experienced increasing difficulty with breathing the last several years because of increasingly severe chronic obstructive pulmonary disease (COPD). His hospital records revealed multiple hospitalizations for bouts of pneumonia. In addition, Vernon noticed that his exercise tolerance had diminished dramatically over the past year. He fatigued easily and was having increasing difficulty managing the day-to-day chores needed to operate their ranch. He and Rachel were considering moving away from the ranch and allowing their children to assume the day-to-day management duties.

Rachel said that she, too, had been a smoker in her youth but stopped when the first of their three children was born. Except for some aches and pains, Rachel considered herself to be in good health for her age and knew that still she could do a good share of the ranch work. Unfortunately, she was unable to do much heavy lifting because of a persistent back ailment. Rachel knew that if her husband stopped working, she would be unable to manage the ranch alone. Recalling the time when her parents became unable to care for the ranch and asked Vernon and her to take over its management, Rachel figured that the time might have come for them to do the same.

His regular physician assumed Vernon's hospital care the following Monday morning, and I did not see him until months later. Unfortunately, Rachel died unexpectedly in the interim. Along with his significant respiratory disease, Vernon had developed a major depression caused by the death of his wife and soul mate of so many years. To complicate matters, his physician had moved from Sidney. Consequently, he came to see me in my clinic when his breathing problems worsened.

On this occasion Vernon was febrile and deathly short of breath. His lips and fingernail beds were blue suggesting a lack of oxygen, which I confirmed with a rapid test done in the clinic. He was coughing up copious amounts of discolored mucus. When I listened to his chest, I heard nothing more than popping and gurgling sounds that suggested Vernon had pneumonia again. I admitted him to the hospital.

The day after being admitted, Vernon suffered a respiratory arrest and lost consciousness. This event required his being transferred to our intensive care unit where I inserted a breathing tube into his windpipe. I attached Vernon to a mechanical ventilator to keep him alive and started to give him high doses of antibiotics and other medications in an attempt to resolve his pneumonia and to improve his marginal lung function.

Before long, Vernon's son Todd arrived in the intensive care unit. He told me that the other two children would come soon. Todd wanted to know his father's medical status, what we were doing for him, and if we thought his father would survive. Todd informed me that he was the oldest child and the one who would make medical decisions for his father's care. He made sure the nurse in the intensive care unit also was aware that he was the one to make medical decisions for his father.

Vernon improved steadily. After a week or so on a ventilator, the lung infection had subsided dramatically, and I was able to start weaning Vernon from the machine. Finally, after being on the ventilator for about ten days, I stopped the machine and removed the tube from his airway.

Soon thereafter, Vernon and I had several long discussions about his lung condition. With his wife gone, Vernon felt that he did not have much to live for. He made it quite clear to me that if he were to have another similar episode in which his lungs failed him, he absolutely did not want to be placed on the ventilator again. He wanted me to allow him to die.

I documented these discussions in my progress notes in the hospital chart. I also wrote a note to the nurse about Vernon's wishes that she placed on the front of the chart so anyone could see it.

After another day or so in the intensive care unit where the nurses monitored him closely, Vernon was transferred to the general medical floor for continued convalescence and pulmonary rehabilitation care.

A few days later, the medical floor nurse summoned me to Vernon's room just as I was finishing my clinic notes for the day. She reported that he was having increasing respiratory difficulty again and asked me to come to the room promptly because she was having an issue with the family. When I asked the nurse what her issue was, she just said, "Dr. A, we need you over here right now, please."

After hearing those words, I hustled to the hospital. When I arrived in Vernon's room, I noticed that Todd and another man dressed in a suit were in the room with two nurses. I saw the nurse who had phoned me and asked, "What's the problem?"

The nurse said that it looked like Vernon was dying. I agreed with the nurse and reaffirmed that Vernon did not want to be resuscitated again. I showed the nurse the note on the front of the chart and the comments in the progress notes.

The nurse explained to me that she had seen the notes, but, unfortunately, Vernon did not make, nor put in the chart, a copy of a living will, and I did not have him countersign my notes to make them legal. Nonetheless, I asked, "So what's the problem? Vernon does not want to be resuscitated, he asked me personally not to resuscitate him, and I assured him I would not. I intend to abide by his wishes."

When I said this, Todd spoke up and reaffirmed his responsibility as being his father's medical power of attorney. He introduced the man next to him as the family attorney. Todd informed me that since his father did not have a living will in the chart or any signed document stating his desire not to be resuscitated, then it was his responsibility to do what he thought was best when his father could make decisions for himself no longer.

I asked Todd to tell me exactly what he meant.

The attorney spoke up and said, "The family demands that you, as Vernon's personal physician, use 'any and all means' at your disposal to keep him alive. The hospital, without a formal document declaring Vernon's wishes, is obligated by law to do everything in its power to care for Vernon." The attorney went on to tell us that if we did not use all available means at our disposal to treat Vernon, he personally would file a civil lawsuit against the hospital and me within days of Vernon's death.

I found myself in quite a predicament. I promised my patient that I would not resuscitate him, but, because of a quirk in the law and in the chart documentation, his son Todd now had absolute control over my patient's destiny.

While Vernon was still breathing on his own, as quickly and as accurately as I could, I notified the hospital administrator of my predicament. The administrator told me to do whatever the son requested. He said the hospital and I would deal with any consequences later.

Soon after this discussion, Vernon lost consciousness. Todd demanded as the medical power of attorney for his father that we place his Vernon back on the ventilator. I felt I had no choice but to comply with the son's demand.

The nurses and I transferred Vernon back to the intensive care unit where, again, I inserted a tube into his airway and connected him to the mechanical ventilator. After I had written orders for the nurses to manage the ventilator and had asked the hospital's pulmonary care aides to provide intensive respiratory cleansing maneuvers frequently during the night, I left the hospital.

The next morning when I arrived in the intensive care unit, Vernon was awake. He glared at me with a wild-eyed stare. He shook his head side to side indicating that he did not want to be on the ventilator again.

I spoke to Vernon. When I was assured that he understood what I was telling him, I informed him that his son had threatened the hospital and me with legal action if we did not reconnect him to the ventilator. I told Vernon that I knew it was against his wishes, but since some paperwork was not completed for the medical record, his son and the family lawyer said they had the legal right to do what they did. The hospital's attorney agreed with them on purely legal grounds.

Vernon just closed his eyes.

While recuperating but still on a ventilator, Vernon had multiple meetings with a gentleman in a suit. I did not know this man, but I did know that he had some discussions with our hospital administrator. I was not privileged to those conversations.

After less than a week on the ventilator, Vernon was successfully weaned from the machine again. When the airway tube was extracted this time, Vernon motioned toward me with his right index finger to come near him. Because the endotracheal tube had caused some swelling of his vocal cords, Vernon could whisper only barely but said to me, “Doc, I don't blame you. I need to rest now.” He then laid his head back to do so.

Vernon rested for the remainder of the day in the intensive care unit with my intention to transfer him back to the medical floor the next morning.

During this episode on the ventilator, I made sure that Vernon's wishes were in writing, in duplicate, and in the chart with his signature. I made sure that there would be no more miscommunication about his wishes. He would not be resuscitated again, no matter what.

When I arrived at the intensive care unit the following morning, I met Todd and his attorney outside the door. They wanted to know why they had been summoned to the hospital. I informed them that I didn't have a clue.

A few minutes after my arrival, the hospital administrator and the hospital's attorney walked into the intensive care unit along with the gentleman who had been visiting with Vernon in the intensive care unit. After short greetings for the morning, they sat down on chairs away from Vernon's bed.

Additionally, one of the local sheriff's deputies came by and stood by the intensive care unit door. I wondered to myself, "What the heck is going on?"

The ICU nurse informed me that Vernon had not done well through the night. She reported that he had refused all respiratory treatments after he was taken off the ventilator. She had not called me during the night to report Vernon's denial of care since now that he had a living will in the chart, he did not want to be resuscitated again, and he made it clear to everyone in the hospital that he really wanted to die on his own terms.

I reassured the nurse that I was not upset with her and thanked her for allowing me to get a good night's sleep. Then I went to Vernon's bedside and asked how he was doing. He said he was doing as poorly as should be expected for someone who had refused our good care. He then sat up a bit, looked around the room, and whispered with a raspy voice, "Looks like everybody's here."

Vernon then looked at his son who was sitting nearby against the wall next to his lawyer. Pointing a finger at his son, he said, "Todd, I gave you the responsibility to take care of me like I wished, and you did not do it. For that I am truly upset." He then stared at the attorney and said, "You encouraged Todd to do something you knew was against my wishes. Consider yourself fired." Vernon then introduced the other man in the room in a suit as the family's new attorney.

Vernon mumbled a few words that I could not understand, but the nurse standing next to me said it sounded like he were saying a prayer to his wife Rachel.

Again staring at Todd Vernon said, "You did not want to let me die which was against my wishes. Now, you are going to sit there and watch me die because that is my wish. If you do not watch me die, you will receive no inheritance."

Todd and his lawyer seemed to be stunned. Todd looked at the floor and said quietly, "Dad, whatever you want." Vernon then said, "That is good," and lay back on his hospital bed to rest. It was as if Vernon had willed himself to die right then because his breathing became more labored almost instantly. Within another half-hour, he was near death and lost consciousness.

Vernon's new lawyer pulled out a piece of paper from his suit jacket, looked at Todd, and read, "I want you to suffer now watching me die, and I want you to see me suffer now and forever, Dad."

It seemed like a very long time before Vernon took his last breath and the heart monitor showed no heart activity, but it was probably only fifteen minutes or so before I pronounced Vernon dead. I looked at Todd and his attorney but did not say a word. I asked the nurse to notify the funeral home and thanked Vernon's new attorney for his attendance.

The new attorney walked over toward Todd, looked him in the eye, and said, "You are responsible for your attorney's fees for this charade. Your father wants you and your family to move from the ranch within one week. Otherwise, you will be charged with criminal trespassing. The sheriff will make sure that you comply with this request. Oh, by the way, your father took you out of his will and you will inherit nothing. Have a good day."

I thought to myself, "Vernon made his own justice. What a courageous man! Good for him." I then walked to the doctor's lounge to get dressed for the morning's surgeries.

You Can't Take It with You

I was on duty as a faculty member with family medicine residents in the intensive care unit one morning when the pulmonologist on duty asked our team if we would be interested in following a very interesting case with him. Without hesitation after hearing "interesting case," we agreed.

When the doctor pointed to one of his patients with severe respiratory disease lying in a bed in the intensive care unit, we could see from a distance that the man was having considerable difficulty breathing. The doctor informed us that he would be placing the man on a ventilator soon because his patient had terminal pulmonary disease. The patient had been on a ventilator multiple times in the past, and the doctor told us his patient really wanted to die.

One of the resident physicians asked the pulmonologist why he was going to put a man on a ventilator when he wanted to die. In response, the doctor explained to us that he and his patient had reached a mutual agreement regarding his ventilator treatment: a maximum of three days. If after that time the patient could not breathe on his own, the doctor was to pull the plug and let him die.

Another resident physician asked if that agreement was not a violation of the hospital's intensive care unit policy which stipulated any patient in the intensive care unit had to receive full care, no matter what. The doctor agreed and continued to tell us there were extenuating circumstances with this case. He informed us that the man had a girlfriend to whom he wanted to leave all of his possessions, and it was going to take his lawyer a day or two to make the arrangements for the man to leave everything to his girlfriend legally before his death. The pulmonologist noted that with the man's current state of health, it could be foreseen he would not survive three more days without ventilator support.

That morning, the pulmonologist placed a tube in his patient's windpipe and connected him to a mechanical ventilator. The doctor encouraged the resident physicians to monitor the man's progress and to observe how the intensive care unit nursing staff managed a patient on a ventilator. He encouraged the residents to ask as many questions as they wished.

For two days we observed the man and the care he received. During the afternoon of the second day, a woman came to visit him. This woman was perhaps twenty years his junior, and I surmised that she was the man's girlfriend. I overheard some of the conversation between these two people. The woman spoke to our patient while he replied by writing on a tablet. The gist of the conversation was that the man knew his days were numbered, the two of them could not be together much longer, and he wanted her to have all his worldly assets. In addition, if she received all of his assets as gifts before he died, he would have no assets to pay any more hospital bills. He figured the hospital was good for it after all the time and money he had put into the place over the years with his previous illnesses. The woman cried while they talked, and when the man got very tired, she left the intensive care unit.

On the third day when the ventilator was supposed to be turned off, a group of people came to the intensive care unit together. Included in this group were the hospital administrator, a hospital attorney, and the hospital chaplain. Our medical team assumed the group was there to watch the man when the ventilator was stopped and to validate his death. As it turned out they were in the intensive care unit to abort any procedures to discontinue the ventilator. Apparently, in his medical records the man did not have a will, a living will, or a medical power of attorney. The doctor's notes in the chart apparently were not adequate for the hospital and their attorneys to allow the man to die on his own terms. Consequently, the ventilator was continued another day.

On the morning of the fourth day, the hospital chaplain came to the intensive care unit to visit with the man. We assumed that since the lack of documentation for the man's final wishes was holding up the discontinuation of the ventilator care, then surely someone could have made the documents available for the man to sign. Our team was confused.

Later in the day, a middle-aged woman walked into the intensive care unit accompanied by the chaplain and the hospital administrator. Apparently, this woman was the man's wife. Our team did not know that he was married and nobody seemed to know how she knew her husband was in the hospital. Apparently, the pair had been estranged and lived apart for almost twenty years, but they never divorced. The woman possessed a medical power of attorney and a will signed by her husband years before when they were together. Legally, these documents evidently trumped all others. This woman let everybody know that she was the person calling the shots with her husband's care.

The woman and the pulmonologist had a meeting regarding his plans for her husband. The doctor presented the original plan for discontinuing the mechanical ventilator and told the woman that her husband's lungs were so bad there was no hope for him to survive off the ventilator, and the patient knew his prognosis.

After this meeting, the woman announced that she would return in the morning with her lawyer. Until then, she ordered that her husband was to remain on the ventilator.

The doctor, who had already consulted the hospital's legal team, concurred. Afterward the pulmonologist confided to our team that he had gotten himself into something that no one would ever have anticipated.

The next morning the wife arrived in the ICU with her attorney to find that her husband had been sedated and lapsed into a coma. After a short talk with the pulmonologist, she commanded the doctor, "Turn the damn thing off." There were several people in attendance at the time including the hospital chaplain.

After asking the intensive care nurse to turn off the power to the ventilator, the pulmonologist removed the ventilation tube from his patient's airway. The doctor then said, "Now that's that." The man's heart stopped a short time later. Within an hour or so, workers from a local funeral home had removed his body.

Several days after the man died, the pulmonologist relayed to our team the rest of the story after his patient's death. Apparently, the man did have an old will that gave everything to his wife, who apparently thought that after years of bitterness with her husband she finally had a windfall with his death. His assets were few but included a pickup truck, a small boat, and a small trailer home. The wife did not anticipate, however, that by accepting her husband's assets she also accepted his liabilities, which included many unpaid debts and a hospital bill well over one hundred thousand dollars. These were now her debts.

We speculated that our patient had notified his wife of his illness and wondered if he had this scenario planned the whole time. The hospital would get paid eventually, he said his goodbyes to his girlfriend, and his wife finally had the responsibility and the power she always desired.

Old Dog, New Trick

A powder made from the bark and the leaves of the willow tree is documented in the historical records during the time of Hippocrates, who lived some time between 460 B.C. and 370 B.C. This powder apparently was used to help treat fevers, headaches, and pains.[56, 57, 58]

It took another 2200 years or more for curious men in Europe during the early 1800s to discover and isolate the compound in the willow plants that relieved pain. The compound was named Salicin. By the mid-1850s Salicin was further purified into a product called salicylic acid, which worked well to relieve pain and reduce fevers. Unfortunately, the chemical's use was limited because of its prominent adverse side effect of irritating the stomach.

Soon thereafter a much improved, stomach friendly formulation of salicylic acid was invented by using a new buffering process. The new chemical was called acetylsalicylic acid (ASA). Unfortunately, the inventor abandoned his discovery around 1860.

At the dawn of the twentieth century a chemist working for the Bayer Company in Germany rediscovered the formula for acetylsalicylic acid. This scientist, Felix Hoffman, administered the product to his father who was suffering from arthritis. After his father reported good pain relief after consuming the chemical, Mr. Hoffman persuaded his employer to market this new wonder drug. Bayer named the product aspirin. Thereafter, aspirin was produced in various forms and became a mainstay for treating arthritis, pain, and fever throughout the world and made Bayer enormous profits.

By the late 1960s aspirin was discovered to have an additional effect of being an anti-clotting or anticoagulant agent. How aspirin affected the body's clotting mechanism was unknown at the time, but its effects were determined to take effect within moments of the drug's ingestion and lasted for three days or more.

I attended a seminar in the early 1980s where one of the lecturers talked about "aspirin, an old dog with a new trick." This physician spoke enthusiastically about the promise of aspirin to become the next miracle heart drug. In this lecture, the original research data suggested that aspirin potentially could provide up to a fifty percent reduction in the incidence of heart attacks and in the number of immediate deaths from heart attacks. This doctor predicted that all future patients suspected of having an acute cardiac event would receive aspirin in emergency situations to eliminate the clot in the coronary artery causing the heart injury.

One morning just a few months after this meeting an ambulance from one of the outlying communities brought a young man complaining of chest pain into our emergency room. Richard Dickensen was only thirty-four years old and complained of having a heavy pressure in his chest. On his arrival the nurse and I noticed immediately that Mr. Dickensen was pale, sweaty, and short of breath. His blood pressure was low and his pulse was elevated. Our hospital staff quickly instituted the current emergency advanced cardiac life support protocols (ACLS). A nurse promptly put an oxygen mask onto Richard's face. Another nurse started an intravenous catheter in his arm for medications and fluids. Also, she placed a nitroglycerin tablet under his tongue hopefully to dilate the arteries to his heart. At the same time, the respiratory therapy technician performed an electrocardiogram (ECG).

The electrocardiogram revealed evidence for a heart attack (myocardial infarction) in progress that appeared to extend across a large portion of the front heart muscle.

Instinctively, I asked the nurse if we had any aspirin in the emergency room. When she replied that a bottle of aspirin was routinely stocked in the pharmacy cabinet, I asked her to give Mr. Dickensen two aspirin tablets immediately. The nurse retrieved the pills promptly and had our patient swallow them.

Over the next few minutes the nurses and I noticed that the changes on the electrocardiogram were going away. The injury pattern that we noticed on Richard's arrival almost resolved. I had cared for many patients suffering heart attacks, but never had I seen the electrocardiogram pattern change as quickly as it did this day. Furthermore, Richard's symptoms appeared to improve. His blood pressure stabilized, his shortness of breath decreased, and his chest discomfort abated. Subsequently, we transferred our patient to our intensive care unit.

Because of his young age and the possible severity of Richard's heart attack, I consulted the cardiologist on call in Billings, Montana, to arrange for an emergency transfer. I knew that Richard might require a surgical procedure on his heart blood vessels to improve his long-term survival.

While the air transport team was en route, Richard's lab work returned which revealed evidence for a small heart attack. By now his electrocardiogram appeared almost normal. However, I knew that the disease process in his heart that caused this heart attack was still there. Still I thought that Richard would benefit from a special x-ray of his heart blood vessels to determine the extent of his disease.

The air transport team arrived by the middle of the afternoon, loaded up my patient, and flew to their home base without incident. After an initial evaluation, the cardiologist telephoned to inform me that he was taking Richard immediately into the cardiology suite at the hospital to perform some special x-rays of his heart and blood vessels, a procedure called a coronary angiogram.

The next morning I received a telephone call from a heart surgeon in Billings who informed me that, after my patient's angiogram revealed severe disease in three major arteries to his heart, he and his partner performed a three-vessel bypass graft procedure. The surgeon informed me that my patient was stable and doing well. He said that it would be a few weeks before the cardiologist could determine exactly how much real damage Richard's heart had sustained.

I became convinced then that the aspirin the nurse administered in the emergency room saved Richard's life and hopefully had limited the damage to his heart.

When Richard came home, the doctors had given him a regimen of several medications that included a daily aspirin tablet. After a month or so the cardiologist determined that the injury to Richard's heart had been minimal, and all his medications were discontinued except for his daily aspirin. I believed the cardiologist and I were of similar opinion when it came to the aspirin therapy.

At the age of forty-two Richard suffered another heart attack which required yet another heart surgery. He continued to take an aspirin pill daily along with a new collection of heart medications. This heart attack caused him to restrict his physical activity, but he was still able to work everyday.

A third heart attack occurred about six years later. This time the cardiologist inserted stents into three of Richard's bypass grafts to keep them open. His heart function after the third heart attack was marginal even on his best days.

Another year passed before Richard came into my clinic on a Monday morning complaining of some vague, nagging chest discomfort. We talked about his and his wife's expectations. Richard really did not want to take a bunch of medicines everyday anymore, nor did he like feeling exhausted with minimal activity. In short, he did not want to live the way he had become. Even though he was only forty-nine years old, he was not sure that he wanted to have anything else done to him concerning his heart.

In my view, Richard was depressed. We had a long discussion about his concerns and wishes.

The next day, Tuesday, Richard telephoned to say he had decided to go back to Billings to be evaluated again. His chest discomfort was just nagging him enough mentally so that he couldn't sleep. I arranged for him to be seen by the cardiologist the next day.

I received a telephone call from a cardiologist on Thursday afternoon who informed me that Richard had a stress electrocardiogram and another angiogram performed soon after he had arrived in Billings, and the doctor informed me that Richard's heart vessels looked fine.

Richard's wife telephoned me Friday morning to let me know her husband had died that morning while walking outside to the garage. She graciously thanked me for all my efforts on his behalf.

I immediately called the cardiologist to let him know that despite his report to me that our patient's heart vessels looked fine, Richard died that morning. There was silence on the other end of the phone. The cardiologist said he would review the results of the procedure and send me a report.

The use of aspirin for acute cardiac disease had become a standard of care by the time Richard died. By the year 2000, emergency room guidelines for acute cardiac care promoted giving aspirin immediately. Extensive clinical evidence proved that this old drug when used alone reduced the severity of heart attacks and the number of deaths associated with acute heart attacks by up to twenty-five percent.

Richard died about fifteen years after his first heart attack. He was productive for fourteen of those years, and he lived to watch his children grow up and graduate from high school. I'm convinced that these additional years with his family were possible because Richard received aspirin while he was having chest pain in our emergency room fifteen years before.

Aspirin is now much older and a lot cheaper, but it remains a wonder drug.

A False Test

It was during the 1940s and early 1950s when researchers found a chemical marker in the blood called prostatic acid phosphatase which was elevated in men with prostate cancer. [59] One of these researchers was C. V. Hodges, M.D., one of my professors at the University of Oregon Medical School. Though not a perfect test, the acid phosphatase served as the only chemical marker for prostate cancer until the 1980s.

By the early 1980s a new marker for prostate disease arrived on the scene named the prostate specific antigen (PSA). [60] The PSA proved to be more sensitive for screening for prostate disease and a better indicator of persistent disease than was the acid phosphatase test. Unfortunately, the PSA was not a very good test for estimating the presence of, or the prognosis for, prostate cancer.

By the late 1980s the PSA test was widely promoted as the screening test for prostate cancer; its attributes were highly publicized. Many cancer groups, physician groups, and healthcare establishments endorsed the PSA as a way to eradicate prostate cancer in our lifetime. Soon the PSA test became a popular screening component in health fair blood panels. In the early days of PSA screening, men were told that if the number was less than four, prostate cancer didn't exist; on the other hand, if the number was higher than twenty-five, cancer definitely existed. Many men, including physicians, accepted the result from a PSA test as the determining factor to diagnose prostate cancer and deferred or eliminated the all-important physical examination of the prostate gland. All too often, relying solely upon the PSA test for cancer detection proved shortsighted for both patients and physicians.

Like many so-called advances in medicine, as well as in life, things are usually not as bad as they are reported to be, nor are they as fantastic and absolute as advertised. Such was the case with the PSA test.

Malcolm Hendrickson was a man in his late forties when he came into my office one day in the late 1980s holding his health fair labs in his hand. Malcolm was feeling good about himself on this day because all the numbers on his health fair lab report were within the normal ranges. He wanted me to perform a complete physical examination so he could get more life insurance and brought the insurance forms with him to be completed.

Before coming to my office, his insurance company had authorized for Malcolm to have a chest x-ray and an electrocardiogram done at our local hospital. His chest radiograph was unremarkable. His electrocardiogram was normal too.

My physical examination was absolutely normal, except for the last procedure, a rectal digital examination. To my surprise, I felt a hard, immovable lump on the right lateral side of Malcolm's prostate gland. I told Malcolm that I could not complete the life insurance examination form until he had the prostate mass evaluated further. Malcolm, who was deservedly taken aback by my findings, promptly said okay.

Despite his PSA test score being only 2.5, which by the rules should have meant that my patient had no disease in his prostate gland, I knew otherwise. I explained to Malcolm that the lump in his prostate gland required a biopsy, and I was going to refer him to a urologist. Still shaken by my finding the prostate mass and by my comments, he agreed to see the urologist; what were his options?

Fortunately, a visiting urologist had an outreach clinic scheduled for Sidney in two days so Malcolm did not have to travel far to be examined. I called the specialist, explained to him what I had discovered, and arranged for Malcolm to have a prostate gland biopsy in our hospital.

Several days later, the urologist called me from his outreach clinic to tell me that his digital examination of Malcolm's prostate verified my findings. He told me that he would call me later in the day after the preliminary results of the biopsies were available from the hospital's pathologist.

At the end of my clinic day, I received a telephone call from the urologist who reported that our patient appeared to have a very aggressive appearing cancer of his prostate which required further evaluation and perhaps surgery. The urologist confided to me that he thought the PSA test surely should have been elevated with the aggressiveness of the tumor. He had already scheduled Malcolm for an extensive evaluation in his office the next week.

The urologist telephoned me about a week later to say that he had removed Malcolm's prostate. During the surgery, he determined that the actual cancer mass in the prostate gland was small. Unfortunately, the tumor was located at the edge of the gland next to the bowel and the nearby lymph nodes where, despite its small size, it had already spread to our patient's lymph glands and his liver. He informed me that Malcolm's prognosis was not good.

Doctors are trained to separate themselves from their patients emotionally to maintain their objectivity, but, in Malcolm's case, I could not remain emotionally detached. Here was a man who was in his mid forties with a wife and family, just like me, who had his entire life turned upside down overnight. I knew that Malcolm, his wife, and their combined families were devastated.

I had a hard time dealing with the thought, "What if I were the one with metastatic prostate cancer?"

Following his surgery Malcolm never regained his vigor. After all the testing was completed, it was obvious he had an extensive malignant process that I had detected early, but unfortunately, not early enough. The pathologist told me my patient's prognosis was perhaps a year or two with treatment.

During the next year as Malcolm received radiation therapy and chemotherapy, both he and his wife became depressed, and I knew that antidepressant medications would not help them. Eventually Malcolm required hospice care and died about eighteen months after the day he had received his normal PSA test result and I found the lump in his prostate gland.

By the year 2000 it became apparent that the PSA test was not as good at screening for prostate cancer as many had hoped for or promised. Clinical data revealed that the PSA was a very poor predictor of prostate cancer because many other disorders could raise the level of the PSA score. Supposedly because of political interference, the United States Preventive Services Task Force (USPSTF) waited ten more years or more to report to the public that it did not recommend routine screening of men for prostate cancer with the PSA test alone. The task force determined that the invasive testing and surgeries associated with falsely elevated PSA tests accounted for far more injuries and deaths than would have occurred otherwise with no testing at all. The final determination was that the testing does more harm than good.[61, 62, 63]

As a rule, prostate cancer is a disease of elderly men, and most of these patients die from a disease other than their prostate cancer. Unfortunately, young men with prostate cancer often have a much more aggressive disease and die from their cancer or from complications caused by its treatment.

When medicine entered the twenty-first century, the old acid phosphatase test from the 1950 s had a renewed interest. Early evidence suggested that the PSA and the acid phosphatase tests used together provided perhaps a better way to screen for, follow, and predict the outcome of prostate cancer.

In the future, as prostate cancer care becomes more focused on identifying and managing a shrinking minority of men who might benefit from extensive prostate cancer therapies, the further use of the PSA and the acid phosphatase tests together in this process certainly holds promise. At least we can hope once more.

Help Me Breathe

When in medical school in the early 1970s, I spent much of my extra time in the newborn intensive care unit. Most of the patients in this unit were premature babies with respiratory disease, and the pediatric staff tried tirelessly and mostly in vain to treat babies born with severe respiratory disease, commonly known at the time as hyaline membrane disease. It was thought that a baby's premature lung had a substance in it that prevented the air sacs from expanding when it took its first breaths. Consequently, therapy was aimed at using mechanical ventilators in attempts to maintain breathing long enough for the newborn's body to remove the substance from the lungs. Later on, corticosteroid medications were given to stimulate the body to remove the substance, but the results generally were not good. In the 1970s sick premature babies born before thirty-six weeks gestation usually died from respiratory failure or complications from the ventilator therapy.

As an intern, I helped deliver triplets who were born six weeks prematurely. I remember vividly Dr. Reginald Franks, the pediatrician in the delivery room, evaluating the babies and walking over to the mother to tell her that her babies were just too small to survive and that there was nothing he could do to make them breathe better. I recall the pediatrician telling me, "If they're born early, they either make it or they don't. There's not a lot that we can do about it today. Maybe tomorrow, maybe someday, we'll be able to help them, but not today."

Fortunately, in my early years of practice I did not have to deal with premature infants often. When I did have to care for them, I observed that if the baby did not breathe well at birth, then its chances of surviving were small. When my own son was born in 1979 at thirty-five weeks gestation with a weight of a little over four pounds, he breathed effortlessly. My medical partner who was caring for my son wanted to transfer him to a regional pediatric center. Since I had received considerably more training in caring for newborn infants than my partner, I reassured him that since my son was breathing well, he was going to be okay. I repeated my mentor's comments to my partner, "If they're born early, they either make it or they don't." I told my partner that my son was born prematurely, he was breathing normally, and he was doing well.

One mid morning in late 1991 while I was seeing patients in my clinic, my nurse knocked on my examination door and reported that I was needed in the operating room STAT. She said there was a newborn from a C-section with breathing problems, and they wanted me in the operating room now.

I told the woman I was examining that I had to leave immediately. The patient said that she had heard my nurse, told me to go, and wished me good luck.

As I was rushing out the back door of my clinic toward the hospital, I told my nurse that I would call her when I knew how long I would be detained. One of my receptionists overheard me and called out, "Dr. A, don't come back today. We will reschedule everybody. Good Luck." Unfortunately, my office staff had been through this drill far too many times before.

I ran to the operating room, which I knew took about thirty seconds from my clinic's back door. I had done this drill many times since a new obstetrician had come to town. Upon my arrival in the operating room, I saw a nurse attempting to ventilate a pale, lifeless baby boy with an AMBU bag (an artificial mechanical airway unit). I saw the baby's chest caving in with each respiratory effort and asked the nurse if the baby had taken any breaths on his own. She didn't know.

I grabbed the AMBU bag and started to ventilate the baby. Since my stethoscope was still hanging around my neck, I asked the nurse to apply my stethoscope to the baby's chest. I could hear air moving in each side of the baby's chest each time I squeezed the bag, so I knew that my resuscitation technique was good.

The nurse revealed to me the baby's apgar score was two at one minute and two at five minutes. Normal newborns usually have apgar scores of 6-9 and 7-9 at these time intervals. An apgar score of two essentially told me that all this baby had going for it was a heartbeat.

To make the situation more stressful, the anxious obstetrician kept asking me how the baby was doing. All I could tell him was that I didn't know yet.

Ventilating the baby by hand, the nurse and I transferred him in an incubator to our newborn nursery across the hallway. There, with the assistance of the hospital's respiratory therapist, I stabilized the baby's breathing by inserting a tube into his windpipe and connecting him to a mechanical ventilator. Next, I inserted two catheters, one into one of the baby's umbilical cord arteries and the other into the umbilical vein, which would allow me to test his blood and give him fluids and medications.

After these emergency procedures were completed and the newborn seemed stabilized, I had time to evaluate the baby further. By my physical examination, I determined the baby boy's age to be about thirty-four weeks gestation. The obstetrician had performed an elective C-section on his patient six weeks early.

A nurse came into the nursery from the operating room to put the baby's name onto the incubator. His name was Nathaniel.

After completing my emergency maneuvers and secondary assessment, I called Dr. Brian Salvino, the neonatologist in Bismarck, North Dakota, with whom I discussed a newborn transport.

After I related my baby's status, Dr. Salvino told me he would be in Sidney to pick up the baby within two hours. Because of the inclement weather, his team would be using a fixed-wing aircraft instead of the helicopter. He told me that the air flight team would call the hospital when they were en route to give an estimated time of arrival and requested that the ambulance be at the airport to pick him up.

I had the lab perform some initial blood work. The radiology department completed a chest x-ray, which revealed the classic ground glass appearance that characteristically was seen with the respiratory distress syndrome of newborn infants. Thankfully, I was able to maintain Nathaniel on the ventilator without any complications until Dr. Salvino arrived in our nursery with his assistant.

After a brief greeting, the doctor examined the baby, the ventilator settings, the lab reports, and the chest radiographs. He concurred with my diagnosis of prematurity at thirty-four weeks with respiratory distress of the newborn. Dr. Salvino then said he had something new to show me. He pulled out a container of a milky looking fluid that he called artificial surfactant [64, 65, 66] and explained to me that he'd been waiting for it to become available for years. He reported that the preliminary results in his newborn intensive care unit for improving babies with respiratory distress were encouraging.

He filled a syringe full of this white stuff and injected it down the endotracheal tube into our little patient's lungs. Afterward he disconnected Nathaniel from the ventilator and turned him carefully in all directions over just a few seconds while, at the same time, patting gently over his chest to spread the milky substance throughout the tubes in the lungs. He then reconnected our little patient to the ventilator.

Dr. Salvino informed me the baby would receive another treatment in a few hours and then again about twelve hours later. Depending on how he did, Nathaniel may or may not receive a fourth dose. Since the product was so new, no one knew exactly how much to give.

About this time, the obstetrician came into the nursery ranting and raving. He demanded that I tell him exactly how the baby was doing. He proclaimed to us that it wasn't his fault. Dr. Salvino politely stepped in front of me to talk to the obstetrician and simply said, "The baby is six weeks early. We're busy." The obstetrician stormed out of the nursery yelling all the way down the hallway.

Dr. Salvino, once he was convinced that our baby was as stable as he was going to be, made sure the mom had a chance to see her baby boy and bid us a pleasant good day. He placed Nathaniel carefully into his transport incubator with the help of his assistant, loaded our little patient into the ambulance, and took off toward Bismarck a few minutes later. Dr. Salvino said he would call when he arrived at his hospital; he promised to keep me updated on our baby's progress.

By the next morning, our little boy was breathing markedly better according to Dr. Salvino, and by the end of the week, he was almost breathing by himself. At the end of ten days, baby Nathaniel was taken off the ventilator but remained in the newborn intensive care unit until he was big enough to go home with his parents.

In the 1950s and 1960s, respiratory disease of the newborn, misleadingly named hyaline membrane disease, was the nation's most common cause of infant death. The most famous victim was the infant son of President John and Jacqueline Kennedy who died in August 1963, two days after being born about six weeks prematurely.

Dr. Mary Ellen Avery[67] as a pediatric resident at Johns Hopkins University in the mid-1950s watched many premature newborn babies struggle to breathe and astutely observed that if the babies died, they usually did so within the first few days of life. If they survived these first few days, the respiratory problems seemed to vanish for no known reason.

Dr. Avery also observed that the babies who died of hyaline membrane disease had no residual air in their lungs at autopsy. It seemed to her that the lungs of babies that struggled to breathe were unable to retain air; she did not know why. In 1959, Dr. Avery and her associate, Dr. Jere Mead, reported after a considerable amount of study that hyaline membrane disease was caused not by the presence of something in the lungs but rather by the absence of something. The lungs of babies who died of hyaline membrane disease lacked a substance they called surfactant, which lines the tubes and air sacs in normal lungs. They coined the term respiratory distress syndrome (RDS) of the newborn.

Thereafter, discoveries about the proteins that comprised the substance called surfactant advanced rapidly. In 1980, a Japanese physician injected an artificial surfactant made from cows into the lungs of babies with RDS; all the babies did well. Multiple varieties of surfactant from different manufacturers were FDA approved by 1990.

In the 1950s, respiratory distress syndrome of newborns claimed between ten and fifteen thousand babies annually in the United States and was the number one cause for infant mortality. By 2010, with the widespread use of lung surfactants, fewer than six hundred babies died from this disease, and deaths from RDS dropped down to the tenth spot on the most common causes of death list.[68, 69]

Nathaniel's mom brought her baby to my clinic when he was about seven weeks old; he now looked like a perfectly healthy, full-term infant. Had I not known better, I would have said Nathaniel's short life had been unremarkable. I could speculate only what might have happened if he had not received the artificial surfactant promptly after his birth.

Nathaniel grew up to be a robust, intelligent young man who graduated near the top of his high school class.

Three Women

As computer technology developed, the quality of the mammography images improved dramatically to the point that evidence for tumors smaller than a few millimeters in size could be recognized. Evaluating these minuscule mammography changes required a breast tissue biopsy that was obtained either through a needle or, more commonly, a formal surgical procedure.

Quite often the pathology diagnosis on these small pieces of tissue was either benign or a low-grade, noninvasive, slow growing tumor confined to the milk ducts called DCIS (Ductal Carcinoma In Situ). [70] To complicate matters, the evaluation of these small samples for cancer cells was extraordinarily difficult for the pathologist to interpret, which resulted in a significant percentage of abnormal positive tests and many unnecessary courses of treatment for breast cancer patients. [71, 72]

Before the early 1980s, the diagnosis of DCIS was rare because the lesions were so small and were detectable only by mammography. With the ever-enhanced resolution of the mammography images over the next thirty years, however, these very small breast lesions became detectable. Doctors felt obligated to treat all early DCIS cancers even if there was only a small chance for them to become malignant and kill the woman. During the next three decades the incidence of invasive breast cancer remained relatively stable while the reported incidence of DCIS increased eight fold, mostly because of aggressive mammography.[73, 74]

Over the years I had the opportunity to care for multiple women who had been diagnosed with breast cancer. When I explained the pathology reports of DCIS to my patients and mentioned the word cancer, the patient often became anxious or panicked. Anytime after the original diagnosis was made the woman became labeled as a cancer survivor even though her chance of dying from the breast tumor may have been small to nonexistent all along.

Following are short case stories of three women with this disease.

I met Delores in our hospital's emergency room one Saturday in 1979. She was a seventy-year-old woman who had noticed some bumps on her chest wall for a few months and, since she and her husband were already in town on business, came into the emergency room to see what the lesions were.

My examination of her chest wall revealed that Delores had bilateral mastectomy scars. Doctors at the Mayo Clinic had removed her breasts about fifteen years before, and, according to both Delores and her husband, the doctors told them that she was free of breast cancer forever.

Now this woman had multiple small, rock-hard bumps along each of her surgical scars together with enlarged, hard lymph glands in her armpits. I knew she had a recurrence of her cancer.

By good luck, the hospital's pathologist, Joe Lasater, M.D., was nearby in his lab, and I asked him to examine Delores' skin lesions for a second opinion. After looking at the lesions, he asked that I biopsy one of them, and he would prepare the material to evaluate under his microscope.

After I retrieved a piece of tissue from Delores' chest wall, I took it to the pathology lab. Before he did anything, Joe told me the lesions were definitely cancer and most likely a continuation of her original breast cancer. He told me, as he had done before, that the natural history of breast cancer is fifteen to twenty years. Joe noted that doctors who advised their patients that they were cured or were survivors after just one year or even five years just didn't know the natural history of the disease. He reiterated that breast cancer was mostly an older woman's disease, and, despite the media hype, very few young women died from the disease. [75, 76, 77, 78]

The tissue sample confirmed a breast cancer that did not appear to be aggressive when evaluated microscopically, and I relayed the report to Delores and her husband. She was devastated and while crying kept whimpering, "They said I was cured." I reassured her that she had lived with her cancer for fifteen years, the tumor did not appear to be aggressive, and the chances were good that she would not die from the tumor. Delores was not relieved. The pair talked about her situation and decided to travel to the Mayo Clinic the next week for an evaluation.

Later I obtained Delores' medical records from the Mayo Clinic and learned that the doctors performed more surgery to remove the skin lesions and the enlarged lymph glands. Radiation and chemotherapy followed. The doctors did not repeat their initial mistake by telling Delores she was cured but instead informed her that she was now a fifteen-year cancer survivor. According to her medical records, the diagnosis from her first breast biopsy fifteen years before was DCIS.

About fifteen years later at the age of eighty-five, Delores suffered a stroke and died in our nursing home. Her breast cancer lesions had returned to the scars on her chest the year before. She had been a breast cancer survivor for thirty years.

She outlived her husband by ten years.

Marsha was a forty-five-year-old mother of four when a screening mammogram found a single spot that looked suspicious. The radiologist recommended and performed a needle biopsy, which produced a small, isolated piece of tissue that was DCIS positive. The size of the lesion was a mere two millimeters in diameter.

Upon hearing the pathology report, Marsha took the news calmly. Her husband, however, was overcome with grief and started to cry uncontrollably. He wondered if his wife was going to die and leave him with a house full of children.

I discussed the nature of DCIS with the couple, and after I talked about the possible treatment options for his wife, the husband wanted to do everything immediately to rid her of *any* cancer. I referred Marsha to an oncologist at a local outreach clinic. The doctor advised Marsha that her chance of dying from her breast cancer was only about five percent. With surgery and radiation, that chance improved to about four percent, and with additional chemotherapy for a year or so, the chance decreased to about three percent. The husband insisted that everything be done for his wife. The doctor arranged for Marsha to undergo the standard regimen of surgery, in this case a lumpectomy, followed by radiation and a course of chemotherapy.

While Marsha was undergoing treatment, her friends held fundraisers, prayer gatherings, and started a support group in her honor. Being a private person, she was overwhelmed and embarrassed by the attention.

As I expected with her type of cancer diagnosis, Marsha did well. Despite being continuously ill for almost a year from her treatments and having treatment associated adverse side effects that lasted for years, she resumed her life as before. When she was feeling well after her treatments, Marsha revealed to me that if the topic of her breasts never came up again, she would be pleased. She was unsure if she would undergo chemotherapy again even if her breast cancer returned.

I last saw Marsha when she was celebrating her fifteenth year of being a cancer survivor.

Olga was an eighty-five-year-old woman I met for the first time in the nursing home while a female resident physician and I were performing monthly evaluations on a colleague's patients. Olga had a long list of medical issues, but as she told us, "I'll be eighty-six soon. I can't complain about my life. At my age, what will be will be."

During my examination of Olga's heart and lungs, I noticed that each of her breasts had visible lumps about the size of plums on the overlying skin. On examination, the lumps were hard, non-tender, and not movable. There were enlarged, hard lymph glands in her armpits also, and I knew that Olga had well advanced breast cancer.

When my female resident saw the lumps, she panicked. The young doctor became quite anxious and told me that we had to get Olga evaluated by a surgeon pronto.

When I asked why she thought a surgeon should be called, the young doctor replied, "To remove those lumps because I think they're cancer."

Agreeing with the young doctor that the lumps were probably cancerous, I asked her if she thought Olga could survive a double mastectomy. The resident did not know, but she told me that if the breasts were hers, she would have as much of the cancer removed as possible.

I suggested we talk with our patient about what she wanted. The young doctor agreed that our patient had the final say when it came to deciding about any treatment.

I told Olga that I was reasonably sure she had cancer in both her breasts and wondered if she wanted me to do anything about it.

Olga replied that the breast cancer was her old friend. She said a doctor found spots in her breasts with a routine breast x-ray when she was about sixty years old. After a biopsy was done, her old doctor at the time discouraged her from having any treatment and convinced her that she would die most likely from something else. With a big smile Olga said, "And here I am. Old Doc Harvey was right."

Olga told us that a young surgeon, who was wet behind the ears, had seen her a couple years before and wanted to remove both her breasts. She got a second opinion from an older, more experienced surgeon who said he wouldn't touch her with a ten-foot scalpel. This doctor explained to her that he did not think she could survive the operation. She had no pain, she felt good, and she still could knit caps for the newborns at the hospital. She didn't need anything else.

That weekend I was able to find some of Olga's old medical records. Her initial breast biopsy diagnosis was DCIS.

At eighty-five Olga was a twenty-five year cancer survivor, and still counting.

She died three years later from heart failure.

Something New

Medical school was to begin in Portland, Oregon, the first part of September immediately after Labor Day. In mid-to-late August, just like all the first-year medical students, I was scrambling to find a place to live. Since I had essentially no money, it was imperative for me to find housing that was reasonably close to the University and affordable. Another student from Montana and I found a home in northeast Portland that was close to the freeway which allowed us easy access to the University's medical school. Together, we figured we could share vehicle costs as well as living expenses.

During our housing search, I talked with several Portland residents who informed me that Portland, Oregon, had two seasons: the summer season, and the rainy season. August was the end of the summer, and Labor Day marked the beginning of the rainy season. Little did I know how accurate their predictions were. The day after Labor Day the sky became cloudy and the rain started to fall. By the end of December, Portland had received about twice as much rain as Montana normally received in an entire year. I do not remember seeing the sun from Labor Day until Christmas.

Local residents also did not explain how Oregon drivers handled, or should I say mishandled, their cars when the weather became inclement. It appeared to me that the harder it rained, the faster the drivers drove on the freeways. One morning I awoke up to find a small amount of snow on my car. In Montana we would have called this a skiff. However, in Portland, Oregon, this was a major snowfall. When the temperature was near freezing but not cold enough to snow, Portland experienced freezing rain and freezing ice storms that produced all kinds of havoc with drivers. It was not uncommon for Interstate 80 to have several multi-car pileups at the same time with some of these massive collisions involving sixty or more vehicles. Obviously, during the snowstorms and freezing rainstorms, the freeways closed. In addition closures included schools, hospitals, and city offices, but the University of Oregon Medical School, which was located on the top of one of the highest hills in the city, always remained open, and medical students were expected to be in class on time despite the weather.

Being from Montana and accustomed to finding alternate routes to avert snow banks and other road obstacles in the winter, the weather did not seem to be a problem for me, while some of our classmates from California and Oregon had all sorts of trouble with ice on the roads. I determined that I if I left my home half an hour earlier in the morning and came home an hour or more later after finishing my classes, most of the rush-hour traffic craziness could be averted. Additionally, my roommate and I determined different street routes we could take to bypass all the congested traffic and car wrecks during bad weather and still get to the school on time and back home safely at night.

One evening the weather report predicted a freezing rainstorm for the next day. Road, school, business, and event closures were made well in advance so hopefully people would stay home. Medical students could not stay home, unfortunately. Therefore, before the rain started to freeze on the roads, I decided to install my studded winter tires on the rear wheels of my car. After I had the winter tires out of the trunk and the car jacked up, I removed the left rear wheel. In the process of installing the snow tire, I felt a severe pain in my left lower abdomen. The pain was enough for me to take notice, so I stood up and felt my left lower abdomen with my hand where I found a hard tender lump that was new. I laid flat on my back, and with both hands pushed on the lump until it was gone and the pain subsided. I figured I had just sustained a new hernia rupture and reduced it, my first medical diagnosis and treatment. After installing my winter tires and having no more pain, I went back to my medical studies.

I had no more difficulty with my hernia for least another week until one day as I was playing basketball the lump and the pain in my lower abdomen returned. I figured it was time to get the lump checked out by a surgeon. Subsequently, I made an appointment to be seen by the surgeons who worked at the Multnomah County Hospital. I chose this clinic because when I had talked with upper class students earlier in the year as we were in the process of selecting our rotations, all of them advised me to go to the County Hospital or to the Veterans Hospital as often as I could for the best experiences. Since I was not a veteran and couldn't go to the VA hospital, I chose the county hospital.

On a Friday afternoon during a break from classes I ventured down to the surgery outpatient walk-in clinic. When my name was called, a nurse escorted me into an examination room and asked me to wait for Dr. Thompson, the senior resident in surgery. Within a brief time I heard a knock on the door and in walked a massive man. Standing about six feet six inches tall and weighing probably two hundred fifty pounds, Dr. Jonathan Thompson was indeed a very big surgeon. On my chart he noticed that I was from Montana and informed me that he came from a ranch outside the small town of Antelope, Montana, in the extreme northeastern part of the state.

When the surgeon asked what he could do for me, I related my episodes and explained to him why I thought I had a new hernia. He agreed that my story was consistent for a hernia, but he had to examine me to make sure that's what I had. Consequently, he had me drop my pants to examine my abdomen. Initially, he could not feel an abnormality. Dr. Thompson had me perform all sorts of maneuvers to strain my abdomen to try to make the hernia appear, but none of them worked. Appearing perplexed, Dr. Thompson just said, "Hmm?" and asked me to stay put because he wanted to have the professor examine me. He then exited the room.

Soon thereafter, Dr. Thompson returned with a diminutive man who he introduced as Dr. Tuck. The name tag on the doctor's coat read, "Jack Tuck, M.D. associate professor of surgery." Dr. Tuck was essentially the physical opposite of Dr. Thompson. He was at the most five feet six inches tall, quite thin, and had much smaller hands. After short introductions and the resident physician mentioning that I was another person from Montana, the faculty physician examined me. He too was unsure if I had a hernia, but he said, "He's a smart young man, the story's right, so my gut feeling is that he's got one."

The doctors talked for a short time about a good time for me to have surgery. Initially they were discussing having me stay in the hospital for two or three days before the surgery and perhaps five days afterward. When I heard them talking like this, I interrupted and told them that I still had to go to school. I suggested that I had a Friday free in approximately two weeks, and if they could do the surgery on a Friday, then I could go home on Saturday and still be back in school on Monday.

To this suggestion, Dr. Thompson responded that things just were not done that quickly at the Multnomah County Hospital. Patients were placed in a queue and surgeries were done as time and money allowed. He also pointed out that essentially all their patients were indigent who did not mind staying in the hospital for as long as the doctors wanted to keep them because they were warm and well fed.

Dr. Tuck came to my defense and noted that I was a healthy fellow and if all went well there was no reason that I could not go home soon after surgery. He knew it was against protocol, but as long as I had good follow-up, he saw no reason why I could not be discharged as I had suggested. The doctors talked again and finally left the room to have a discussion with the surgery-scheduling nurse. Upon their return Dr. Tuck said the nurse acted as if they were stealing her only child but agreed to our shorter-stay surgery plan. According to Dr. Thompson, we were going to do something extraordinary at the Multnomah County Hospital; they were going try something different.

After classes late Thursday afternoon I went to the county hospital to check in for surgery. Unlike the fancier State Hospital with its private and double rooms, the Multnomah County Hospital had wards of beds. After being admitted to the hospital, I was settled into one of eight beds in a surgical ward about eight o'clock in the evening. Post-surgical patients were resting quietly in six of the other beds. The only patient awake was a man in a bed across the room from me and wanted to chat for a while. Since I had nothing else to do, I listened.

The man told me that I didn't look like the usual customers that came to the county hospital. He asked me what I did. When I told him I was a medical student, he wondered why I wasn't in the fancy State Hospital across the street. He informed me that only the poor folks came to the county hospital.

I informed the man that I was a poor medical student, I thought I would get the best experience in the county hospital, and I chose to come to the county hospital.

The man, who looked as if he had been in a fight with his face scraped and bruised and a couple of his front teeth knocked out, wanted to know what kind of surgery I was expecting to have. I told him that the doctors were planning to perform a hernia repair on me the next morning and that I should be out of the hospital by Saturday. To this the man laughed and said, "Hey kid, good luck with that." He then went on to tell me that he came in for hernia repair three weeks before and was still in the hospital. He cautioned me not to get my hopes up for going home early. I had to admit that his comments bothered me. I certainly couldn't stay in the hospital for three weeks and miss that many classes.

Dr. Thompson came in to visit me about 9 p.m. He informed me that I was first on the list in the morning and that someone would come to get me about 0630. He asked me if I had any concerns or questions, and when I had none, said he would see me in the operating room in the morning.

I was escorted to the operating room a little bit after six o'clock the next morning. I saw my two surgeons and two anesthesiologists who informed me that they had decided to give me a regional anesthesia, a spinal block, to expedite my surgery. They promised me that I could remain awake and watch the surgery on a mirror they had situated above me. I thanked them.

After the spinal anesthetic was instilled and produced a good result, one of the anesthesia doctors asked me to watch the mirror. That was the last I remembered until severe pain in my back awakened me from a stupor and someone was asking me if I was okay. When I finally awakened with my face down in the pillow, I saw the blurry outline of my classmate John sitting next to my bed talking. He kept asking me if I was okay. I must have responded to him somehow because he said that he was worried about me and that I looked like hell. I must have asked about the time because he told me it was four o'clock in the afternoon. Hearing this, my brain engaged for some reason; I knew that I was supposed to be in my room and awake by ten o'clock in the morning.

The anesthetic fog lifted slowly from my mind allowing me to talk with my classmate about what happened to me. All he knew was that he had been sitting by me for close to four hours, and I had been dead asleep the entire time. The pain in my back was excruciating, and I complained about it to John. He said I had been asleep twisted like a pretzel the whole time and told me to look at my feet.

Twisting my face from the pillow to see the end of the bed, I found my toes pointing up. I tried to move them but couldn't, so with John's help, I got untwisted which instantly relieved the back pain. My legs were still tingling as the spinal block wore off but were not useable yet. Over the next few minutes my mind cleared, and once he was assured I was going to be okay, John left.

Soon after John departed, a large, powerfully built female nurse came to check on me. She said it was about time for me to wake up because it was almost time for supper. I told the nurse that I was a bit nauseous and wasn't really hungry. She responded by telling me that if I expected to be discharged in the morning, then she had better see me eat something for supper. Before I could say another word, the woman went to see other patients on our ward and within a short time left the room.

When the nurse had passed the ward's door, I heard the patient across the room say, "Hey laddie. What did I tell ya? There is no way in hell you're getting out of here tomorrow." I was starting to worry that he was right.

About seven o'clock the large nurse brought in my supper. All the other patients had eaten their meals two hours before at a time when I was just waking up and in no condition to eat. She told me that I was only getting a late supper because I was a medical student and she was being nice to me. In a threatening tone, the nurse demanded that she had better see some food gone from my tray by eight o'clock when her shift ended, or else.

Not wanting to eat, but still wanting to leave in the morning, I figured I had better eat something. I took the lids off the dishes on the tray to find the most amazing post surgical meal of all time: a cold, dried piece of liver, four cold Brussels sprouts, a hard dry piece of toast, a dollop of runny coleslaw, a container of warm milk, and a peanut butter cookie. I started gagging the instant I saw and smelled the liver.

From across the room, the man who now figured he was my best buddy on the surgical ward asked if their was a problem. He had heard the nurse's ultimatum and wondered if he could help me out. I told him that liver and Brussels sprouts literally made me sick, and except for the peanut butter cookie, I didn't think I could keep down anything else on the tray. The man told me to eat what I could and he would eat the rest. I removed the cookie and offered him the rest.

The man eased himself out of his bed and slowly walked over to my bed for my food. Before he took the tray he said he would show me his incision if I showed him mine. My wound was still covered by a bandage and there wasn't much to see, but I said okay. I showed the man my abdomen with its new clean bandage over my hernia repair site. The patient then dropped his hospital gown pants to the floor and said, "Look what happened to me." He had bruises extending from his umbilical button to his knees with his scrotum the size of a grapefruit. As I was gawking at him, the man cautioned me to beware because my doctors were the same ones who had operated on him. He then took my tray and went back to his bed. Fortunately, he devoured the food and had my tray returned to my bedside by the time the nurse returned. Before leaving, she just smiled and bid me good night.

Before I could go to sleep, the man wanted to talk some more. He wanted to bet me on what I would get for breakfast. I thought it was a silly bet because I had not ordered a breakfast. He said that my not knowing should make the bet so much more interesting. When I asked him what he wanted to bet for, he offered to bet for the part of my breakfast that I did not want. After seeing my supper, I hardly could wait for breakfast. I made the bet and asked him to tell me would be on my breakfast tray. He replied: a hardboiled egg that is so rubbery you could bounce it off the walls without bruising it; toast so hard you can't take a bite out of it without it crumbling into pieces; frozen, rock hard butter; oatmeal so sticky that it won't fall out of the bowl when held upside down; cold coffee; hot milk; and a scorched pancake topped with frozen syrup. I knew nothing could be that bad and told him he had a bet.

Morning vital signs were taken about 6:30 a.m. followed almost immediately by breakfast. While the dietary aides dispersed the trays to the patients, the man called across the ward to make sure I remembered our bet, and I acknowledged that I had. When I removed the lid from the top of my tray, I saw everything exactly as my fellow patient had described the night before and was amazed. I asked him how he knew what was going to be on my tray. He replied that the breakfasts at the county hospital had been the same for the past three weeks, so he knew he couldn't lose. The scorched pancake was all I could eat; my ward companion got the rest and relished every bite.

The two surgeons came in about ten o'clock escorted by the heavyset nurse who I soon discovered was the nursing supervisor for surgery. After the doctors had removed my bandage and checked my incision, Dr. Tuck told me that my diagnosis was correct and I had a routine hernia repair. I asked if I was still scheduled to leave that day. Dr. Tuck said he saw no reason to keep me unless I wanted to stay. I admitted to them that I was concerned that I might end up like the other surgical patient on the ward who had his hernia repaired.

Dr. Thompson told me not to listen to that guy and asked me if the patient told me what really happened to him? I admitted that he had not, and both doctors grinned. They asked the nurse to relay the man's saga.

She explained that the patient was an alcoholic with two hernias. The doctors watched him for three days in the hospital to make sure he would not have alcoholic withdrawals after his surgery. The evening after his operations the man developed alcohol related delirium (DTs), saw strange creatures coming after him, and tried to get away by jumping out of his bed with the side rails up and his arms restrained. The nursing staff found him about half an hour later thrashing about while being high centered on the bed's side rail bar. This activity destroyed his surgical repairs, contused his genitals, produced a large blood clot inside his scrotum, and made him appear that someone had beaten him. The nurse added that if I were not a heavy drinker then I should not need to worry. The doctors told me I was cleared for discharge and arranged for me to see them in the surgery clinic in one week. Before departing, the nurse smiled and whispered that she knew who really ate my supper.

The anesthesiology doctors came in about half an hour later. I learned that the younger doctor was a first year resident and the one with the gray temples was the professor. The younger doctor said he had to apologize for the anesthetic he had given me the day before. He confessed that he gave too much medicine for the spinal block which made the anesthetic extend too far up my spinal cord. This in turn caused me to have some breathing problems. In his effort to sedate me, the doctor said he gave me too much medicine which totally turned off my respiration drive. He had to ventilate me manually for two hours before I could breathe by myself. The young doctor knew that the surgeons wanted to see if I could be ready to leave the hospital by the end of the day of my surgery, but it didn't happen. Speaking positively, the elder physician told me that I was never in any danger; it just took twenty-four hours for the anesthesia to clear my system instead of the two hours they had planned.

My roommate John took me home that Saturday afternoon where I relaxed the remainder of the weekend and prepared for class Monday morning just as planned.

I saw Dr. Thompson for a follow up visit a week later. After he examined me and told me I was good to go, the doctor said that the short stay surgery idea went well except for the anesthesia glitch and thought that there might be more use for it someday if the bugs could be worked out of the system. Forty years later the vast majority of surgeries were done outside hospitals in outpatient surgery centers where the patients came from their homes, had the surgical procedures performed, and returned to their homes the same day.

SENIOR MOMENTS

"I've learned that people will forget what you said,
people will forget what you did,
but people will never forget how you made them feel"

Maya Angelou

Charge Me Double

Outside on the examination room door was an attached written note from my nurse that said, "Wants to talk to you." This type of notation usually meant that I could be in for a psychiatric session or something similar. I took a deep breath and entered the examination room.

I immediately recognized Camilla, a woman in her late eighties who was the matriarch of a local ranching family. I sat down on a stool and asked Camilla what problem I could help her with. Camilla just sat there thinking and staring at the wall. She said, "I know it was important, but I forgot what I was going to tell you. I drove all the way in from the ranch to tell you something; now I can't remember what it was."

I tried to jog Camilla's memory by asking her if she hurt anywhere or if she had been sick in any way. She felt fine, and she knew I was well aware that she was healthy as a horse. Next I asked her if there were any problems with anyone in her family. Camilla said that, as far she knew, all the kids, grandkids, and great grandkids were all feeling good and not having any major problems.

Since other patients were waiting to see me, I asked Camilla if it would be all right if I gave her some time to think about what she may have forgotten. In the meantime, I could see some of the waiting patients. She thought that would be okay.

A short time later I went in to visit Camilla. She confessed she just could not remember why she wanted to see me and offered that she would go home for the day. If she remembered what she wanted to say, she would call me. Camilla then said, "This getting old is for the birds. I can't remember a damn thing!"

About this time one of my office personnel brought in a piece of paper another client had found on the floor in our reception area. My receptionist looked at the paper, thought that it might belong to Camilla, and brought the crumpled piece of paper to Camilla.

Camilla looked at the note on the paper and said, "Doc, now I know what I wanted to tell you. Do you remember Jacqueline my granddaughter whom you delivered almost twenty years ago?" I confessed that I did not remember her granddaughter's birth per se, but I did remember her granddaughter Jacqueline when she was in high school. "Well," Camilla explained, "little Jackie's going to get married to some fellow she met in college." I congratulated this grandmother on her good news and thanked her for sharing with me.

As Camilla was about to leave the exam room, I told to her that there would be no charge for her visit today. But Camilla did not stop. Now that she started to remember things, she continued to tell me about her granddaughter, her fiancé, how they were doing in school, what they were studying, her children, the other grandkids, and so on for another fifteen minutes or more.

Suddenly Camilla paused, thought for a few moments, and said, "Now aren't I a foolish old woman. Here I am taking up your valuable time for something so silly, and I couldn't even remember what it was about anyhow." She insisted that I charge her for an office visit.

To this I responded that I enjoyed our visit and there still would be no charge. To this Camilla replied, "I will hear none of it. I can afford it, so charge me." I handed the routing slip with a NO CHARGE written on it to my receptionist.

As she made her way to the reception area, Camilla said, "Come to think of it, you should charge me double because of the amount of your time I used up and the trouble I caused." My receptionist glanced at me with a puzzled look and mouthed the words, "What do you want me to do?"

With Camilla standing by the payment window where she could hear me, I asked my receptionist to bill Medicare for double the amount.

Camilla was happy.

Obviously, I knew double pay for a bill that was zero was still zero. My receptionist just raised her eyebrows and smiled.

Speed Bump

One weekday morning I was evaluating one of my patients in the nursing home during my monthly rounds when there was a commotion outside the door. It sounded to me as if someone had fallen. It was the kind of sound that one does not want to hear in a nursing home for fear that something could have happened to one of the residents.

While my patient waited for me in her room, I walked to the doorway to see what was going on. I was the first to arrive at the scene of the accident. In the middle of the floor a short distance down the hallway was an elderly man lying prone with his cane still in his right hand and his spectacles lying nearby. He was not complaining of any pain, but he was letting out a long string of swear words.

When I made my way up the hallway, I could see the man was another one of my patients, Clarence Bellingham. Several members of the nursing staff arrived moments later.

Mr. Bellingham was a retired rancher who had very poor vision because of macular degeneration, arthritic hips that required him to walk slowly with a cane, and intermittent confusion. He was mad as heck and continued to swear, but he appeared to be no worse for wear after the spill. I asked Mr. Bellingham why he was lying on the floor.

After a few more swear words, he yelled, "Can't you see I fell down?"

Next, I asked him if he was hurt anywhere to which he replied, "Hell no. Just my pride."

When I asked Mr. Bellingham if he could tell me what happened to him, he yelled out, "Whoever put that speed bump in his hallway ought to be shot. This is the third time this month I've tripped on the damn thing."

I looked at the floor and saw no speed bump. However, there was a dark line across the hallway made with tile. Apparently the architects in their wisdom during a recent remodeling job had decided to break the monotony of the hallway by inserting a few dark lines in the tile floor. They did not realize that elderly people with poor vision and shuffling gaits, like Mr. Bellingham, might think the line was something to step over. They could fail to make it over the line.

After the nurse and I determined that our patient was indeed not injured, we managed to get Mr. Bellingham upright and walking down the hall again escorted by a nursing aide. He continued to swear all the way down the hall to his room.

I asked the charge nurse what she thought could be done to make the hallway safer. Apparently Mr. Bellingham was not the only one who had tripped over the speed bump. She informed me that the engineering department was planning to replace the tiles making the line in the near future.

"I hope it gets done sooner than later," I muttered to myself and suggested this to the nurse.

I then resumed my patient visitations, which required another two hours. When I finished, I noticed that the speed bump floor tiles had been painted over with a quick drying spray paint that matched the color of the surrounding floor tiles. The nurse told me that the paint was a temporary fix because a permanent repair would take days to complete.

Before leaving the building, I asked Mr. Bellingham to go for a walk with me down the hallway with a story that I wanted to make sure he was okay before I left for the day. Mr. Bellingham didn't even notice the painted repair on the floor as he shuffled right over the previous speed bump without any problem.

I turned around and gave the charge nurse a thumbs-up for a job done well.

The Starting Line

Having agreed to fill in for a physician in a rural eastern Montana community when he had to leave his practice abruptly for a family emergency, I arrived in the afternoon on the Sunday before I was to begin working. To become acquainted with the medical facilities, I made my way to the hospital, which, like many Montana hospitals, was a combined hospital and nursing home complex.

After I introduced myself to the nursing staff, I walked up and down the halls to see where everything was in the hospital and nursing home building. When I made my first pass down one of two nursing home hallways, I noticed an elderly woman standing patiently in the middle of the hallway with her walker. I greeted her for the evening, and she returned a similar salutation.

Approximately ten minutes later, I walked down the same hallway where the same elderly woman supported by her walker continued to stand patiently in the middle of the hallway. I asked her if I could be of assistance. The woman indicated that she was waiting in line for supper and pointed to the floor where a dark square had been made with colored floor tiles.

I had not been in the facility very long, yet I knew that the dining area was at the other end of the corridor. I asked the elderly woman if I could escort her to the dining area, but she insisted that she was going to be first in line to have supper. I could hear voices coming from the cafeteria so I knew that the evening meal was already being served. Again, I encouraged the woman to allow me to assist her to the dining area, and again, she insisted that she did not want to lose her place in the food line.

Somewhat puzzled, I walked over to one of the young nursing aides in the facility and directed her attention toward the woman standing in the middle of the hallway. I informed the aide that the elderly patient was waiting at the spot on the floor for supper.

The young employee laughed, told me she could take care of the problem, walked up to the elderly woman and said, "Abigail, why are you standing here?" Abigail replied, "I wanted to be first in line for supper tonight, so I'm standing here at the starting line."

With a youthful giggle, the young nursing aide responded, "Abigail, you got the lines confused again. This is the finish line, not the starting line. The starting line is at the other end of the hall by the cafeteria door."

As the teenager looked at me, she asked Abigail if she would like to be escorted to supper by the new doctor in town.

Standing less than five feet tall and steadying herself on her walker, Abigail looked up at me and pronounced, “Times a wasting young man. It's time to eat.”

I had the pleasure of escorting Abigail with her walker to the cafeteria for the evening’s meal. Unfortunately this evening she was the last one off the starting line.

Deaf as a Post

Crawford Collingsworth was about eighty-five years old when one of his daughters escorted him into my clinic for an annual checkup. The daughter revealed that her father was extremely hard of hearing and had been so for years. She confessed that buying his expensive hearing aids had been a flat out waste of his money. The daughter insisted her dad could read only her lips. Therefore, she would act as my interpreter, if I did not mind.

I told her I did not object.

While his daughter spoke, Crawford sat quietly in his chair until his daughter touched him on his shoulder and, while staring directly at his face, she yelled in her high-pitched voice, "Daddy, I'm going to be right here while the doctor checks you. Is that okay?" Crawford nodded affirmatively.

I knew that many cases of hearing deficit were a high frequency sound loss caused by extensive noise trauma to the hearing nerves. I also knew communication could be enhanced by speaking with a louder, lower-toned voice. Therefore, I purposely spoke loudly with a lower-toned voice to Crawford.

He understood my questions and responded appropriately, so I concluded that we did not need the services of his daughter to communicate after all. Upon learning that Crawford had been an avid hunter for scores of years and had served with the artillery corps during World War II, I understood how the nerves to his ears were damaged.

In his eighties, Crawford took no medications. He last visited a physician about ten years before, and Crawford told me that the previous doctor said he was in good shape for his age.

Crawford had no physical complaints except for his hearing problem and an occasional leg cramp. He had obtained his hearing aids about five years before when he said they worked pretty good for a short time. He continued to say that for the last year or so the hearing aids had not worked worth a damn. Since her dad and I seemed to be communicating satisfactorily, the daughter left the examination room while I performed my physical examination.

For being in his mid-eighties, Crawford was indeed in good physical condition. About the only things I determined to be abnormal for his age were his poor hearing, copious hard, dry wax in his ear canals, and arthritic changes in his finger joints. After I removed the wax from his ear canals, Crawford said that he could hear a lot better already.

While checking his hearing aids, I observed that the ventilation tube in both devices was full of the same hard wax, and I removed it with a pipe cleaner rod that the local audiologist had given me. I asked Crawford when he last changed the batteries in his hearing aids. He didn't remember ever changing the batteries. "Was I supposed to?" he asked.

Hearing this, I took Crawford's hearing aids to the local audiology office located nearby in our clinic building, and asked the technician to clean thoroughly the units and install new batteries. The technician assured me the procedure would take just a few minutes and that she would deliver the devices to my office when she was done.

I walked back to my office to finish examining Crawford. In my absence, my nurse had obtained a blood sample for some routine screening tests, and she informed us that because of the upcoming weekend holiday the results would not be available for a couple of days. Crawford offered to return to the clinic whenever we wanted.

With the wax removed from his ears, Crawford again mentioned that his hearing was better already.

The technician returned with the hearing aids. She explained to us that the tubes were dirty, the batteries were dead, and somehow both units were turned off. I thought to myself, "No wonder he couldn't hear. The hearing aids didn't work."

After the audiology technician showed Crawford how to change the batteries and how to turn on his hearing aids, she placed the units into his ears. Crawford said that he could hear a pin drop. With his newly found hearing, Crawford said he was just tickled pink. He repeated that he would be pleased to return to get his lab results in a couple of days.

As promised, Crawford came back several days later with his daughter. While they were in the reception area, I saw Crawford's daughter speaking loudly to his face so he could read her lips just as before. I concluded that Crawford's hearing must have been worse than I thought, and our efforts had been fruitless. Crawford had his daughter stay in our reception area while he came back to the examination room.

As I entered the examination room, Crawford burst out, "Doc, before you say anything, I gotta tell ya that the hearing aids work great."

I asked why his daughter was yelling at him.

Sporting a big cheesy smile, Crawford replied, "I turned them off this morning. I haven't told anybody. It's been pretty interesting being able to sit around the house, looking dumb, and listening to what people say about each other and me." With a tone of indignation, Crawford quipped, "I'm about ready to change my will."

I just smiled in amusement before I presented Crawford with his normal lab test results. Crawford Collingsworth lived another decade probably turning his hearing aids off and on.

Can't See

Clients in assisted living facilities, as a rule, are able to care for themselves with minimal assistance from the professional caregivers whose jobs are to manage their clients' medications, provide their meals, and provide them a safe living environment. I was visiting a patient in our local assisted living facility one day when I passed an open doorway with an elderly woman sitting in a wheelchair.

She called out to me and asked if I had seen her spectacles.

I replied that I had not seen any spectacles lying around.

The woman appeared somewhat distraught and said that she couldn't go to the dining area without her glasses; she couldn't see very well. She continued to tell me that she had looked all over and had failed to find her spectacles.

I offered to take a look in her room for glasses, if she wanted.

The elderly woman replied that she would appreciate that very much saying, "Do you realize how hard and frustrating it is for an old person like me to find their glasses without wearing their glasses?" The way she made the comment made me chuckle. I went in to look around her apartment, which was not very large. I checked every flat surface, behind every piece of furniture, on the floor, and in the bathroom to no avail.

After I completed my search, I asked the woman if she had been anyplace else that day. Replying that she had been all over the building, she lamented that her glasses could be anywhere. She then told me that one of the young girls who worked at the assisted-living facility had tried to find her glasses in her room and had failed also. Apparently, the aide was searching the rest of the facility where this woman supposedly had been earlier that day. The elderly woman then developed a look of despair.

When I pulled up a chair beside her wheelchair to console her, I noticed that she had a scarf on her head that was holding back the hair from her face. I also noticed that the scarf was not lying smoothly on her head but appeared to have something under it. I asked her if I could remove her scarf.

She wondered what on earth for?

I explained that her head was the only place I had not looked for her spectacles.

The elderly woman removed her scarf and, lo and behold, there sat the lost pair of glasses straddled on top of her head. I removed them and noticed they were as thick as coke bottles, a validation that her vision was quite poor. I handed the pair of glasses to her.

Donning her newly found glasses, the elderly woman commented, "Oh my, I must have put them there when I was washing my face before going down to the dining room, and I forgot. I always put my scarf on without looking in the mirror. Aren't I the silly old biddy?" The elderly woman thanked me for my efforts as she readied herself to go to the dining room.

Before departing, I suggested that with such poor vision she might consider having a spare pair of glasses in her room just in case her regular glasses got misplaced again. I told her that it was obviously difficult for her to find her glasses without wearing her glasses. She smiled and nodded in agreement.

Before leaving, just to be sure she didn't forget again, I watched the woman write a note to herself to get another pair of glasses for her room. Her note read, "Get new glasses to find the old glasses!" I bid the woman a good day.

On the way out of the building, I conveyed my story to the nurse on duty who in turn could tell the nursing aide that the lost spectacles had been rediscovered. The nurse promised to make sure the woman obtained a new pair of glasses before her old pair was lost again.

My Daily

I had been in Sidney, Montana, for just a short time before I became acquainted with Lars Federstrom. Lars, a diminutive widower in his early seventies with a long history of depression, had incurred multiple abdominal operations over the years. By all accounts, he was well known by to the doctors and pharmacists who had ever been in Sidney.

With an obsession with his bowel function, Lars had been evaluated multiple times by many doctors in many places. The answers were always the same: depression, laxative abuse, and loneliness.

About three a.m. one Saturday morning, the emergency room nurse telephoned my home. Upon my answering, she informed me that Lars Federstrom was in the emergency room again, and he needed to see me right away. It was urgent.

I asked the nurse if Lars appeared ill, and she said that he looked totally fine and was in no distress. He just needed to see me.

I asked the nurse if he realized it was only three o'clock in the morning? She just replied that Mr. Federstrom was waiting patiently for me in the emergency room.

Begrudgingly, I got dressed and drove the four miles from my home to the hospital. I walked into the emergency room to see Lars sitting comfortably in a chair. After offering a good morning welcome to the nurse and Mr. Federstrom, I asked what I could do for him.

Lars looked me in the eye and said emphatically, "Doc, I haven't had my daily yet."

I replied that I wasn't sure what a daily was.

Looking perturbed and becoming quite animated, Lars said, "You know, my daily. The old two over one, old number TWO, the big T W O, the big boomer, the big B M." He asked if he had jogged my memory.

I almost started laughing at his antics, but without thinking and with dead seriousness I said, "Well, Mr. Federstrom, it's now almost four o'clock in the morning, and you know what, I haven't had mine yet either."

After hearing this, Lars looked at the clock, put on his coat, and said, "I guess I can wait." He then walked out of the emergency room without muttering another word. The nurse and I just looked at each other and laughed. What else could we do?

SPECIAL PEOPLE

"There are only two ways to live your life.
One is as though nothing is a miracle.
The other is as though everything is a miracle."

Albert Einstein

One Old Cowboy

It was summer in Sidney, Montana. The grain harvest was well underway, and it was county fair time in the Lower Yellowstone River Valley. By tradition, a rodeo was held for several days during the fair, and I soon learned that rodeos meant there would be considerable work to be done in the hospital emergency room repairing cowboys.

I had spent most of the afternoon in the emergency room repairing rodeo cowboys in one way or another. While I was placing scores of stitches in a bull rider's face, the emergency room nurse called out and said that she had another cowboy to be seen. She told me that she would put this patient in the trauma room because the other beds were full. I assured the nurse that I would see the patient when I completed suturing my patient's wounds.

The nurse suggested that I did not have to be in a hurry because the patient was not in any hurry and not acutely ill. I then watched the nurse push an elderly man sitting in a wheelchair into the trauma room. Seeing that the man had a bandage around his head and an arm was in a sling, I thought to myself, "He's a rodeo cowboy?"

After I completed repairing the wounds on the bull rider's face and arranged for him to be seen to have the sutures removed in a few days, I walked into the trauma room. The elderly man, who I guessed was about eighty years old, was still sitting patiently in a wheelchair. He appeared to be comfortable. I introduced myself to my new patient.

The patient replied, "My name is Walter Otto, and I'm from Circle, Montana. My friends just call me Otto."

I told Mr. Otto that I noticed that he appeared to have a nasty cut on his face above his eye, and he must have hurt his shoulder because it was in a sling. I asked him if I was correct in my assessment.

He said, "My name is Walter, not Mr. Otto, but most folks just call me Otto." He continued to tell me that he and a heifer got a little bit crosswise that morning. He chuckled a bit, and then said, "I believe the heifer won this bout." He told me that while moving cattle out of a corral that morning, a heifer got feisty and slammed him against the corral. Walter explained in detail what happened to him in the corral and how he was no match for a thousand pound cow. Walter (I used his first name.) figured his left arm got hurt at the shoulder when he hit the ground. He also figured the laceration on his face happened when his head hit one of the metal crossbars on the corral.

I asked Walter where he wanted me to start. He suggested that I start with his head because it didn't hurt as much as his arm. I countered with evaluating his shoulder first explaining that then I could take x-rays of the shoulder if I needed them. While the x-rays were being processed, I could repair the cut on his face. Walter thought that was pretty fair thinking.

After this short talk, I examined his injured arm. He had pain with any motion of any part of the arm. Additionally he had point tenderness over the shoulder. I decided that x-rays were indeed indicated and had the nurse escort him to the radiology department.

I had just finished repairing lacerations on yet another cowboy when Walter returned from the radiology department holding the films of his shoulder on his lap. I reviewed the pictures and saw no acute fractures. However, I noticed that there were multiple changes related to old injuries and arthritis in the left shoulder. I explained the pictures to Walter and mentioned that his shoulder had been injured in the past. Walter confirmed that he had been a pretty good cowboy in his youth and had taken some serious lumps a few times.

Since Walter's shoulder was not fractured, I left his arm in the sling and started to evaluate his facial cut. After cleaning the area and removing all the dirt and grass, I sutured the wound without incident.

Sometime during this episode a middle-aged to elderly woman entered the trauma room. She introduced herself as Mrs. Otto. For the most part, she stood aside and just observed the activities in the emergency room. When it was time for Walter to depart the hospital, he must have decided it was time to chat a bit. Walter spoke up and asked, "Doc, ya got a minute to shoot the bull?"

Since there were no new patients waiting in the emergency room, I told him, "Sure." Walter said, "Young man, did you know that I was a land baron out by Circle?"

I replied, "No sir. How much land do you have?"

After thinking for a few moments, Walter continued with, "I've got a lot of land. It's either sixteen sections or sixty-four sections, I just can't remember anymore. I do know that when I stand on the hill by my house it's as far as I can see in all directions." At this point his wife interjected, "Otto, you know you've got cataracts. You can't see the hood of the car. Besides, the hill behind the house is only twenty feet tall. You can't see anything from the top of that darn hill." Walter countered with, "I still own a lot of land." He asked me if I had ever seen any of the large tractors that had four-wheel-drive and eight tires. I told Walter that I had seen these tractors, but they usually were out in the dry land farming areas. My neighbor told me that these machines were too large for the irrigated farming that was done in the Lower Yellowstone Valley around Sidney.

Walter said, "Well, I've got four of them. I drive them all."

Mrs. Otto interrupted, "Walter, you know that's not true. You're just filling this young man's head full of nonsense. You haven't driven those big tractors in some time. You know that the boys and the grandsons are the ones who drive those big tractors now." Mrs. Otto went on to tell me that a few years before, Walter had thought that the field of sprouting spring wheat was full of weeds. Thinking he would clean up the weeds, he hooked up one of the big four-wheel-drive tractors to a forty-foot-wide heavy disk and continued to disk up the weeds. After this incident, the sons did not allow Walter to drive the big tractors without an escort.

Walter insisted that he still drove tractors around his place. Mrs. Otto explained that her sons had fenced off a ten-acre plot that was Walter's plot only. They reconditioned an old John Deere B tractor that has only two cylinders and could not be more than ten to fifteen horsepower. The boys attached the small tractor to a ten-foot-wide cultivator implement. Walter was allowed to rip up this piece of earth to his heart's content.

As they were preparing to leave, I asked the pair how long they had been married. Walter told me they'd been married a long time. Mrs. Otto rebutted that they had been married just a short time. She was Walter's third wife. His first two wives had died. She said they did not get married until she was sixty-two years old and he was about seventy-five.

When I asked Mrs. Otto when her first husband died, she replied that Walter was her first. When I inquired why she waited so long to get married the first time, Mrs. Otto replied, "I wanted to make sure that I couldn't get pregnant." She laughed.

The nurse applied a large bulky bandage onto the sutured wound on Walter's face. She reassured him that if he got contrary with another heifer, the big bandage would protect his head a little bit. Walter laughed. Mrs. Otto told us that she would make sure that her husband did not play with the cows for a few days.

I told Walter that I wanted him to keep the sling on his arm for a few more days and then start rehabilitating his shoulder with some easy exercises. I then gave him a list of exercises with illustrations that he could do at home to prevent his arthritic shoulder from becoming immobile from lack of use. Walter pronounced that he did not need the exercises. He stated emphatically that he worked on a farm, and he exercised his whole body every day.

Mrs. Otto informed me that there was a nurse nearby their home who could remove the stitches from Walter's face at the appropriate time and wondered if that would be okay with me. She didn't want to make the long journey back into town just to get some stitches removed. I told her that I thought that was a good idea. I suggested to Mrs. Otto that the nurse could call me if she had any concerns or questions.

To my surprise, Walter and his wife came to my office a few days later to have his sutures removed. When I asked Walter why he came all the way into town just to remove the sutures when his neighbor nurse could have done the job just as well, he asked, "Hey Doc, you got some time to shoot the bull? I've got some stuff to tell ya." After I removed the sutures from Walter's face, we shot the bull for another half hour or so. Mrs. Otto stayed around to keep her husband's stories close to accurate.

I had the opportunity to care for Walter, his wife, and members of four generations of his family for another twenty-four years. Over the years Walter and I shot the bull a few more times. I even learned to call him "Otto."

He died a year or two after his one-hundredth birthday.

Doctor Carl

During medical school I had a marvelous experience during my surgical rotations. The surgical residents and professors seemed to be truly interested in making sure that I was prepared from a surgical experience standpoint to go on to my next level of training. With this as my background, I had high hopes and expectations during my internship that I would receive the training that I would need to perform surgical procedures competently when I started private practice.

Dr. Raymond Rossman, the director of medical education for our internship program, brought me into his office before my surgical rotation. He informed me that I would be spending the next eight weeks with Dr. Samuel Carl. Dr. Rossman explained to me that Dr. Carl trained at the Mayo Clinic and was the senior surgeon on the hospital's surgical staff and at his multi-specialty clinic. In his opinion, Dr. Carl was one of his best preceptors, and he assured me that I could expect an outstanding experience. In addition, the doctor cautioned me that Dr. Carl was tough and demanding. In Dr. Rossman's mind, Dr. Carl was the most demanding preceptor on the medical staff. He wished me luck.

Surgery was going to be my next rotation immediately after my training in the intensive care unit. I was on call in the intensive care unit the weekend before I started my surgical rotation. When I had some free time that Sunday evening, I went to the surgical floor to ask the floor nurses what was expected of me the next morning when I made clinical rounds with Dr. Carl. I met with the charge nurse on the general surgical floor during the afternoon. She advised me that Dr. Carl made patient rounds at precisely 5:15 a.m. and warned me not to be late.

Even though I had been up most of the night in the intensive care unit, I was able to sleep for approximately one hour before I made my way to the surgical floor. I arrived at the surgical nursing station at 5 a.m. to see the night nurses still on duty. They explained to me that Dr. Carl preferred to have patient rounds with the night nurses so nothing got lost regarding his patients' conditions during the nurses' change-of-shift reports.

The charge nurse instructed me where to stand when Dr. Carl came to look at the charts. She told me that when he got up to see his patients, I would walk on his left side, one half step behind him. She described how the nurses would walk precisely three steps behind Dr. Carl and would carry his patients' charts. This was how it had been done at the Mayo Clinic when he trained, and this was the way he had been carrying out his morning patient rounds for over thirty-five years. I thought to myself, "Talk about being compulsive."

At precisely 5:15 a.m. Dr. Carl stepped out of the elevator and walked toward the nursing station. He was a short elderly man who stood only five feet six inches tall or less. I introduced myself to Dr. Carl.

He never looked up from the charts that were stacked on the counter. He just said, "Have you looked at the charts?" I replied, "No sir, I just got to the floor myself." Dr. Carl responded gruffly, "That's your job."

He then asked the charge nurse if there had been any problems with his patients during the evening. After the nurse reported that there had been no significant adverse events during the night, Dr. Carl started to evaluate each patient's chart in a particular sequence. When he had completed his inspection of the medical records, he stood up and said, "Let's go."

With those words he stood up and started walking down the hallway to his first patient's room. The charge nurse nodded her head toward me and pointed toward his left shoulder as she had instructed me previously. The nursing train started with the charge nurse whose job was to write any order that Dr. Carl may give in the chart. Two additional nurses followed behind the charge nurse holding the patient charts in a precise manner with the charts cradled in the left arm.

Upon entering the patient's room, Dr. Carl walked to the sink and washed his hands with a bar of Dove soap. (Later on one of the nurses told me that the soap had to be Dove soap and Dove soap only.) Dr. Carl then walked to the bedside where he had to awaken his patient. It was 5:30 a.m. The doctor asked this very groggy woman some vague questions about how she felt. Obviously, since she was barely awake and had recently received an injection of a narcotic pain medicine, the patient had no real complaints.

Dr. Carl removed her surgical bandage and evaluated her wound. With his index finger he motioned for the charge nurse to bring the patient's chart to him. In a low mumbling tone he gave the charge nurse some orders for his patient, which she promptly transcribed onto the order sheet in the chart. After reviewing the nurse's orders, he initialed the chart entry.

Again he went to the sink to wash his hands. This time Dr. Carl demonstrated to me the appropriate way to wash hands before and after evaluating each patient. He had me show my hand washing technique to him. When I started to wipe my hands with a towel, the surgeon admonished me and said, "You always pat your hands dry. You never rub them dry. You always pat your hands dry. Understood?" When I demonstrated that I could pat my hands dry correctly, I received nods of approval from the charge nurse and Dr. Carl.

Without further delay the doctor said, "Next patient." This process continued until we had seen approximately ten patients. When all the morning rounds work was done, Dr. Carl looked at his watch, looked at me, and said, "The knife falls at seven a.m. sharp. Let's get to surgery."

While in the elevator Dr. Carl told me that I would be the intern assistant for him and his two surgical partners. He expected all of their patients to have a complete history and physical examination performed by me the evening before surgery. The history and physical was to be dictated and on the chart by seven a.m. Furthermore, I was to write a legible, brief summary of the essential parts of the history and physical in the medical record just in case something happened with the transcription process. In addition, Dr. Carl said that I was expected to research the surgical procedures that I would be assisting with before the procedure. These duties were not negotiable.

I do not remember the surgeries Dr. Carl and I performed that first morning. However, between surgical cases, I ventured up to see the patients we had seen earlier that morning to determine if there really were any new problems. As I suspected, most of the patients did not recall our morning visitation. Indeed, most of the patients had questions for Dr. Carl that I could not answer. The best that I could do was to write down their questions and present them to him between surgical cases.

Dr. Carl and I finished with his surgeries about one o'clock in the afternoon. He told me he was going to the clinic and that I was responsible for the immediate postoperative care of the new surgical patients. When I presented my questions to him for the post-surgical patients that were in the hospital, he told me to look up the answers. As he was leaving the surgical suites, Dr. Carl said that he wouldn't see me until rounds the next morning.

I thought I had time to get some lunch before I went to see my patients on the surgical floor, but one of Dr. Carl's partners had me paged to report to surgery immediately. I had not been told that Dr. Carl's partner, Dr. Johnson, started his surgical day at one o'clock in the afternoon and that I was expected to be in the operating room fifteen minutes early.

Gobbling down a portion of my sandwich on the way to surgery, I arrived just as Dr. Johnson was finishing placing the sterile drapes over the patient. I figured I wasn't too late.

After assisting with several more cases with Dr. Johnson that afternoon, I finally got back to the surgical floor to see my patients about six p.m. The nurse on duty informed me that I had three new patients to evaluate for surgery the next day. Additionally, she had concerns with five post-op patients. I must've looked tired and hungry because the nurse said, "Dr. Ashcraft, there are some snacks in the nurses' station if that would be helpful."

I thanked the nurse and ventured toward the table to review my culinary choices for the night. After a quick snack, I managed to handle the concerns associated with the five surgical patients. Then I continued on to perform the history and physical examinations on the three new surgical patients. While my patients were settling down for a good night's sleep, I was completing the written part of the medical records, writing preoperative orders, and finally completing the dictation that was required for the medical records. I finished my duties just after midnight. Fortunately, I wasn't on night call this evening so I figured I would have time to sleep for a few hours before we made patient rounds again at 5:15 a.m. sharp

This process continued for the next three weeks. During that time I figured I had spent approximately one hundred twenty hours per week evaluating and caring for the patients of Dr. Carl and his associates. Also during this time I was allowed to do little, if anything, surgically in the operating room except to cut an occasional knot, adjust the surgical lights, and provide wound exposure. In essence, I was working my behind off and getting no actual procedural skills experience. In three weeks I had not even been allowed to insert a single stitch or tie a surgical knot in a patient. I thought to myself that this was not the quality surgical experience that I had hoped for. Certainly to this point my hands-on experience was far less than I had had received in medical school.

I had a discussion with Dr. Rossman, our director of medical education, and requested a transfer to another surgeon. I informed

Dr. Rossman that I was frustrated by my workload and not getting the experience that I thought I needed to become a good primary care physician in a rural community. Dr. Rossman told me that no one had ever requested removing Dr. Carl as his or her preceptor. He requested that I give him a few days to see if he could straighten things out with Dr. Carl.

Dr. Rossman called me into his office several days later. He revealed to me a conversation he had had with Dr. Carl and that Dr. Carl was somewhat shaken by my request. Dr. Rossman said Dr. Carl had told him that every morning he conducted teaching rounds from which I should have learned a lot.

I informed Dr. Rossman that Dr. Carl's so-called teaching rounds included trying to wake patients up at 5:15 in the morning, his saying no more than two or three words in each patient's room, and then walking down to surgery without saying a word. I suggested to Dr. Rossman that he talk with the nurses on the surgical floor who took care of Dr. Carl's patients if he thought that my description of the process was inaccurate. He told me that he would check with the nurses.

The next day as I was walking from the surgical suites to the surgical floor I saw Dr. Carl exiting from an elevator. He came up to me and said, "I understand you have issues that I have not addressed." Over the next five minutes or so the surgeon and I had a discussion of my concerns and my expectations from what was left of my surgical rotation. After the discussion, Dr. Carl said he would see what he could do to fix things.

The next morning I received a call from Dr. Rossman asking me to come to his office. He wanted to know if I had had a discussion with Dr. Carl. When I told him that I had met Dr. Carl as he was coming out of the elevator the day before and had a short discussion with him, Dr. Rossman said he had pointedly asked Dr. Carl, "How many times did you insert a stitch or tie a knot before you performed it correctly?"

Dr. Rossman told me that, before Dr. Carl could respond to his question, he informed him that I was putting in over one hundred twenty hours a week taking care of his patients. The least he could do was to allow me to perform some simple surgical procedures. Dr. Rossman said that Dr. Carl agreed with him and promised to see what he could do to adjust things a bit.

This discussion occurred on a Friday afternoon. I was on surgical call for the weekend and did not see Dr. Carl until Monday morning. Our first surgical patient on Monday morning was a middle-aged menopausal female who had developed some irregular bleeding from her uterus. This woman had been referred to Dr. Carl by the woman's internist. As we were scrubbing our hands before surgery, Dr. Carl informed me that I would be performing the dilatation and curettage procedure (D&C) on the woman and asked me how I would perform the procedure.

Since I had performed this procedure multiple times as a medical student, I felt confident that I could do it well. I described to Dr. Carl the procedure as I had done it before. As we made our way into the operating room I noticed that the surgical technicians had already placed sterile drapes around the patient. The anesthetist had administered general anesthesia to the woman, and she was well sedated. Dr. Carl and I both sat down on movable stools in the operating room and assumed our positions at the end of the table to perform the procedure.

Dr. Carl initially located himself directly at the end of the operating table as if he were going to do the procedure. With a quiet voice he announced to the surgical team, "Dr. Ashcraft is going to take this one." He moved aside so I could assume the position of the surgeon.

I performed the procedure flawlessly, even if I do say so myself. I was able to retrieve a significant amount of material from the woman's uterus, which was promptly sent to the pathology lab for a quick preliminary testing and diagnosis. (This is called a frozen section preparation.) We sat and waited in the operating room while the sample was being processed. Nothing was said in the operating room. There was morbid silence.

Ten to fifteen minutes elapsed before we heard a crackling noise on the intercom speaker. A male voice identified himself as the tissue pathologist for the day and said bluntly, "Dr. Carl, your patient has cancer." The doctor asked Dr. Carl if he would be needed anymore for this case. Dr. Carl thanked the doctor and told him that his services were completed for the day. The speaker in the operating room crackled as the pathologist hung up the telephone.

The next thing I knew was that I was flying across the operating room on my wheeled examination stool and crashing into the operating room door. Behind me I heard Dr. Carl scream, "God damn intern. You gave my patient cancer. Get the hell out of my operating room." I heard loud gasps that came from the surgical assistant and the anesthetist. I replied to Dr. Carl, "No sir!" Dr. Carl then cursed at me and yelled, "Well then, help me get her off the table and back to post-op."

After we got the patient transferred onto a gurney and before she was moved to the post anesthesia recovery area, Dr. Carl stormed out of the operating room. While leaving, he said, "Cancel my cases for the day." He then just walked out of the surgical area.

That afternoon Dr. Carl's partner, Dr. Johnson, paged me. When I met with Dr. Johnson in the surgical lounge he told me that he and Dr. Carl had had a discussion about his female patient with uterine cancer. He also said that he had talked with the personnel in the operating room. He apologized for Dr. Carl's behavior and told me that his partner had been under an ungodly amount of stress recently. He explained that Dr. Carl's wife was quite ill and he had been preparing for an important meeting. He also informed me that Dr. Carl would be gone for the rest of the week to attend an educational seminar, and we would be performing a hysterectomy (removing a woman's uterus) on the woman with cancer the following morning.

Dr. Johnson and I performed the hysterectomy without any problems the next morning before we performed five additional operations. Afterward, Dr. Johnson thanked me for my help (something Dr. Carl had never done) and informed me that the other surgeons at the clinic would be evaluating Dr. Carl's post-op patients for the next few days. He asked me to talk with the surgical nursing staff to see who would be making rounds on Dr. Carl's patients. He then proclaimed, "I'm almost sure that we won't be making rounds at five o'clock in the morning."

I learned that Dr. Carl's wife was a patient in the hospital, so early that evening I went to visit with her just to see who would be married to someone like Dr. Carl. I found her asleep in a hospital bed with one of his clinic partners sitting at the bedside. Apparently, the doctors had decided to have someone near her the entire time that he was gone. I learned that she and Dr. Carl were special people in the eyes of many in the Spokane community.

I do not know if Dr. Carl said anything to his colleagues. Yet, after this incident, I was allowed to perform an increasing number of surgical procedures under the guidance not only of Dr. Carl's partners but also under the guidance of other surgeons on the staff. Over the next four weeks, I was allowed to repair hernias and hemorrhoids. I removed gallbladders. I performed various gynecologic surgical procedures, and I removed part of a traumatized colon.

After Dr. Carl returned and resumed his normal routine, he still said very little to me. On his first day back, we performed an abdominal operation that went smoothly. When it was time to close the abdomen, Dr. Carl just turned around and walked out of the operating room. I stood there for a few moments next to this patient with an open abdomen before I asked the surgical nurse, "What do we do now?" The nurse explained to me that Dr. Carl had just given me permission to complete his operation. The nurse told me that she had seen him do that only once before in twenty years. She hinted, "He must think you're doing a pretty good job."

After closing our patient's abdomen and making sure the he was transferred to the anesthesia recovery room in good condition I sought out Dr. Carl. I was told that he had already gone to his clinic, and I had new patients to evaluate for the next day's surgery schedule. Therefore, I made my way to the surgical floor and continued with my usual duties.

The following morning at 5:15 a.m. sharp when Dr. Carl came to the surgical wing to see his patients, I met him before he got to the nurses' station. I thanked him for allowing me to close the patient's abdomen the day before. Dr. Carl stated curtly, "You were ready." He then continued on with his normal routine of morning patient rounds.

For the next three weeks little changed. Dr. Carl carried on his life in medicine as he had done for almost forty years. However, he allowed me more latitude in caring for his patients. One patient in particular was deathly ill with an abdominal abscess that we could not locate since we did not yet have the luxury of CT scans, MRI scans, and other noninvasive diagnostic tools that are available today. We just had to wait until the abscess declared itself one way or another. I was allowed to manage the patient's extremely complex fluid and nutrition problems. After we struggled with this patient's dilemma for about a week, Dr. Carl decided to transfer the patient to the University of Washington Medical School in Seattle.

About ten days later, Dr. Carl received a letter from a surgical professor at the medical school who complimented him on his management of this patient with such an obscure problem. In particular, the professor pointed out to Dr. Carl that the patient surely would not have survived had he not received such aggressive and comprehensive fluid management and nutrition care, which was the care that I had provided.

I left Dr. Carl's surgical team a short time after this episode. He wouldn't even shake my hand. Apparently, this was his way of remaining emotionally disengaged. About a week later, Dr. Rossman's secretary summoned me to his office to get my surgical rotation evaluations. All of my reviews from the various surgeons with whom I had worked were good to excellent. Additionally, Dr. Rossman said that Dr. Carl told him that I was one of the best surgical interns he had ever had. Not only was I shocked, but also I was utterly amazed. Unfortunately, I had no time to thank anyone. I was now on to my obstetrics rotation with a woman who was about to deliver a baby.

In retrospect some years later, I concluded that my experience in surgery, although extraordinarily difficult in the beginning, eventually exceeded my expectations and prepared me well for my years ahead practicing medicine in rural Montana.

Sam

It's late in the evening on Monday, December 6, 1976. I was in the hospital emergency room caring for other patients when the emergency room nurse received a telephone call from a woman who said her husband was so dizzy he could not stand up and had been throwing up all day. She asked the nurse to send the ambulance to their home.

After receiving appropriate responses to a routine series of questions, the emergency room nurse told the caller that she would dispatch the ambulance as soon as possible. After telling the woman that she would return a call once the ambulance had departed from the hospital, the nurse paged the ambulance crew and advised them of the patient in distress. She asked me to stay in the emergency room to see this new patient since the weather outside was not good, and I was already in the hospital. That way, she would not have to contact the physician on call and have him drive on the slippery wintry roads. As always, I agreed to stay. After the ambulance crew left the hospital to retrieve the patient, the nurse returned a call to the patient's wife as she had promised.

The ambulance returned within a short time since the sick man and his wife lived in town only a short distance away. The patient was transported into the hospital emergency room on an ambulance cart accompanied by a middle-aged woman who I assumed to be his wife.

While the emergency room nurse was completing paperwork and obtaining our patient's vital signs, I had the opportunity to talk with one of the EMTs about their assessment of the patient. One EMT told me that this man was stiff as a stick at his home. They noticed that he had a pot near his bedside that he had been using when he vomited. Another EMT reported that the man's vital signs were stable throughout their encounter. Additionally, I was informed that he had Parkinson's disease.[79, 80]

I went to see my new patient. He was a pale, diminutive man in his late fifties who appeared to be much older and seemed to have difficulty thinking. This man was frail, weak and soft-spoken, which made his speech almost inaudible. I noticed the classic tremor of Parkinson's disease in both hands. He was able to tell me that his name was Sam Floyd and pointed toward the woman near him and introduced her as his wife Harriet.

After this short introduction, Harriet promptly took over the conversation. Whenever I asked her husband a question, she would give an answer and then would say, “Isn't that right Sam?” To this, Sam always would nod his head in agreement.

When I started asking questions about Sam's medical history, Harriet asked me, “How long are you going to be here?” Thinking that she was talking about this visit in the emergency room, I told the pair I would be there as long as it took me to figure out his problem. Harriet asked me when I was going to move out of town. I informed her that I had moved my family to the Sidney area recently and had no intention of moving, as far as I knew. I mentioned that they had asked me an interesting question and wondered why they thought I would be leaving.

Sam spoke up and asked with a sly smile, “How much time have you got Doc?” I reassured the pair that I would take had as much time as we needed to figure out Sam’s problem. Both of them nodded in agreement, and Sam said, “That sounds good.” Harriet then started to give me Sam's saga with doctors over the previous five years, something I never could have expected.

Sam Floyd and his wife Harriet were longtime residents of Sidney, Montana, in the Lower Yellowstone River Valley. About five years earlier when Sam was about fifty years old, he developed problems with generalized muscle pain and increasing difficulty with thinking that forced him to stop working. After months of trying to figure out his medical problem, Sam's local family physician at the time concluded that he had reached a diagnostic dead-end and referred Sam about nine hundred miles away to the Mayo Clinic in Rochester, Minnesota, for an evaluation by their specialists.

After multiple tests and comprehensive evaluations by many doctors that required several weeks’ time, Sam's doctors at the Mayo Clinic concluded that he had a progressive neurological disorder called Parkinson's disease. The Mayo Clinic physicians started Sam on a medicine called L-dopa and watched him for several days to see how he responded to the new medication. When Sam seemed to be responding appropriately to the medicine without too many adverse side effects, he was discharged from the hospital at the Mayo Clinic. The doctors requested that Sam return in a few months for another evaluation. In the meantime, he was asked to see his local physician who could oversee his transition to his new medications.

Sam returned home to Sidney and started to visit his local

physician frequently. Sam, Harriet, and their local physician were all pleased with the improvement in Sam's mental function and muscle problems while taking the new medicine. Unfortunately, the L-dopa proved to have a significant number of unfortunate side effects, which Sam tolerated only because his physical and mental problems improved.

Just before Sam and Harriet returned to the Mayo Clinic for a follow-up visit, his local physician decided to leave town. This predicament forced Sam and Harriet to choose another personal physician from the several other doctors available in town. After getting opinions from family and friends, Sam and Harriet selected a new personal doctor who, after he had heard Sam's history, was agreeable to see him as a patient. Sam had all his records transferred to his new family doctor.

When Sam and Harriet revisited the Mayo Clinic and after his evaluation was positive, the Mayo doctors informed Sam that they no longer needed to see him for his Parkinson's disease. The Mayo physicians thought his local physician could monitor his medications as well as they could, so no follow-up visits were planned at the Mayo Clinic. The doctors did suggest, however, that a neurologist in Montana follow Sam because a neurologist would be able to modify his medication dosages more efficiently and quicker.

Harriet said they felt as if the doctors at the Mayo Clinic had abandoned them, but they agreed to find another doctor in Montana. As Sam interjected, "What else could we do?"

According to Harriet, the couple returned to Sidney, and soon thereafter, Sam visited with his new local doctor to discuss the evaluation results from the Mayo Clinic. Sam noted at this time their new doctor sincerely seemed to be concerned about his condition and voiced a desire to do whatever he could to make him more comfortable. Even though they all knew that Sam's Parkinson's disease was progressive and not curable, Sam and Harriet were reassured when they knew they had someone locally who was going to help them if Sam had trouble.

About a month went by before Sam consulted a neurologist in Billings, Montana, about two hundred seventy miles away. Harriet reported that the neurologist told them that he made trips to northeastern Montana on a regular basis to see some of his patients. This pleased both of them. The idea that they would have to travel only a short distance to see the neurologist, especially in the winter, was gratifying news.

A few days after this visit to the neurologist, Harriet said she received a phone call from their local physician's office manager who informed Harriet that their office had received Sam's medical records from a neurologist in Billings, Montana. The woman also told her that since they had not informed their local doctor about wanting to see a neurologist in consultation, he would not see either of them as patients ever again. The office manager told Harriet that Sam's records were ready to be picked up that day. Otherwise, the records would be destroyed.

Harriet said she was flabbergasted. They had done nothing wrong. In fact, they had done exactly what the Mayo Clinic doctors had asked them to do. Harriet thought that surely there had been a mistake by somebody somewhere. Without delay, she went to the doctor's office to correct this misunderstanding.

Harriet told me that the office manager was waiting for her when she arrived with Sam's records in an envelope on the counter. Harriet opened the envelope to show the office manager that the Mayo Clinic doctors' records recommended that Sam seek out a neurologist closer to home, which they had done.

Harriet thought this information certainly would correct any misunderstanding and hard feelings. It did not. The office manager told Harriet that her doctor's decision was final, and that was that. The woman handed Harriet the packet of records and said goodbye.

Harriet continued to tell me that she did not go home right away but instead ventured to another doctor's office in town to make an appointment for Sam. When she presented her tale of Sam being refused treatment by the other doctor in town to the new office manager, the woman asked Harriet to wait in the reception area a few moments while she spoke with her doctor. After a few minutes the office manager returned to inform Harriet that her doctor was mad that they had not come to see him first. Therefore, he would not take them as new patients. The office manager was very sorry and wished Harriet good luck in finding a new doctor for Sam.

Harriet was dumbfounded. When she arrived home, she related her discussions with the doctors' employees to Sam. Together they had a long discussion about their options and decided that they would seek medical care outside of Sidney in another nearby town.

After a few days, Harriet located another physician they liked in a nearby community who seemed to care about treating Sam and his Parkinson's disease. This doctor had no problems managing Sam's condition and his medications in conjunction with their neurologist. This physician even gave Sam his home phone number in case he needed him in an emergency. They were convinced that this new doctor had solved their dilemma.

Despite the medications, Sam's condition deteriorated significantly over the next year or so. The neurologist tried more medications with the perpetual admonition that Parkinson's disease was progressive and not curable. The specialist hoped that the new medications would be effective for a long time but nonetheless warned them that he had no idea how well, or if, the new medications would work.

Meanwhile, Sam's new primary care doctor left town abruptly about year later without giving them any notice. Harriet said she found out about the doctor's departure when she tried to make an appointment and received a phone recording advising that the clinic number had been disconnected. Again, Sam and Harriet were searching for a new family doctor.

In the meantime, several days before coming to the emergency room, Sam had visited his neurologist in Billings. The neurologist started Sam on yet another medication on Thursday of that week. On Friday, Harriet received a call from a nurse in the doctor's office in Billings to tell them that the doctor had become severely ill, requiring his immediate retirement from medicine. She told Harriet that Sam would have to find another neurologist, and she was going to send Sam's medical records to them in Sidney so that they could give them to their next neurologist.

Unfortunately, the new medication given to Sam by the retiring neurologist produced substantial adverse side effects, which now brought him to the emergency room. Now Sam was without a neurologist and a family physician. He had progressive Parkinson's disease symptoms with severe side effects from his new medicine. Sam and Harriet did not know where to turn. Now I understood why the pair had wondered how long I would be staying in Sidney. They wanted their doctor merry-go-round to stop; I could not blame them.

After patiently listening to Harriet's extended history, I evaluated Sam. Each time I tendered Sam a question, Harriet would provide an answer. Finally, I asked Harriet to go to the cafeteria and get a drink of water so that I could talk to her husband privately. After some convincing, Harriet left the emergency room with the nurse so that Sam and I could be alone.

After my examination, I concluded that Sam's dizziness was related to his new medication and not to a new illness. Unfortunately, his persistent vomiting had left him dehydrated, and he was going to require a considerable amount of intravenous fluids. I arranged for him to be admitted to our hospital to receive the fluids and to stop his new Parkinson's medicines.

It took several days for Sam to improve to the point where he could go home. During this time, I contacted doctors in the neurology department of the Mayo Clinic and asked them for their advice regarding Sam's medications. The doctors were kind enough to fax me their instruction sheets for the same medications that Sam was taking. With the added help from the local internal medicine specialist, who unfortunately was planning to depart Sidney in a few months, Sam's medications were managed adequately.

Thankfully for Sam and me, his Parkinson's disease remained stable for the next year or so. During this time, I became acquainted with a new neurologist in Billings, Montana, who had trained in England and at the Mayo Clinic and was coming to Billings right out of his training program. I arranged for Sam and Harriet to visit him. Luckily, the pair seemed to get along well with this new doctor. What was more important to Sam and Harriet was that the new doctor informed them he and his family had no intention of leaving Montana.

Over the next fifteen years or so I had the opportunity to care for Sam with his Parkinson's disease in conjunction with the neurologist in Billings. Additionally, I cared for Sam and Harriet when other medical problems emerged. As his Parkinson's progressed, I often checked Sam at his home when he was unable to get out because of bad weather or illness.

When Sam was about seventy, I cared for him in our hospital after he suffered a heart attack and a small stroke near the same time. As usual, Sam took this setback in stride. Harriet, however, was devastated, but her attitude improved dramatically when he left the hospital several weeks later.

Two more years had passed before I admitted Sam to the hospital with a severe infection in his urinary system that had spread to his entire body. At the time I told Harriet that Sam was very ill, and I was not sure how long he would live. Harriet remained at his bedside for several days without going home. Finally, Sam persuaded his wife to go home to get some rest. He convinced her that he had already said his goodbyes, and he was ready to die if that had to be. Harriet reluctantly went home to rest that night.

I was in the hospital this particular evening after I had assisted a woman in childbirth. While I was completing medical records after the baby's delivery, a nurse asked me to come to Sam's room because he looked really bad.

Without delay, I went to Sam's bedside. As I sat by him, he tried to say something to me but was just too weak. Motioning with his hand for me to come closer to his face so I could hear what he had to say, Sam asked me if I thought he was going to die that night. I told him that I thought he would die soon and that I would call Harriet so she could be with him. Sam became a bit agitated and said, "No, Harriet has been through enough."

I asked if there were anything I could do for him to make him more comfortable, and he said that he was having worse pain and would like some medicine for it. I cautioned Sam that he already had received a dose of morphine, and if I gave him more, he may not wake up. I asked if he understood what I was saying. Sam nodded to show me that he understood. I was about to get up from my chair to go to the nurse's station to order some more morphine when Sam grabbed my hand. Again, I asked him if there were something else I could do.

Sam said, "You stayed with me all of these years. You never left me like the other doctors did. You were true to your word after our first visit, and you never left me. I want you to know how grateful I am. Please do not leave me now." I sat down next to Sam's bed and held his hand. I did not have to order more pain medication. Sam died peacefully and quietly about ten minutes later.

After Sam died I telephoned Harriet to let her know that her husband had passed away. Harriet wanted to know if I was with Sam when he died. I assured her that I had been with him at the end. Harriet told me that Sam had wanted it that way. Tearfully, she thanked me for caring for Sam for the past many years. She then hung up the phone.

I had the privilege to care for Harriet for another six years before she died. Each time I saw her she would tell me how appreciative she and Sam had been of my efforts to care for them for all those years, and how I never deserted them. This touched me deeply.

Space Wizard

Glen Stover first came to my clinic in the early 1980s when he was in his mid-twenties. At the time all he wanted was a refill of his medications. Glen's history was that about a year before he had been at the Mayo Clinic for a follow-up examination for a childhood illness. He told me the Mayo Clinic's doctors discovered that he was behaving differently.

The short version of the story was that Glen spent a week or more in the acute care psychiatric hospital in Rochester, Minnesota, where the Mayo Clinic psychiatrists diagnosed him with a chemical imbalance in his brain and started him on two medications. One medicine called Stelazine was for his thinking problems and another medicine called Cogentin was to counteract the many adverse side effects of the Stelazine. Glen swore that the Mayo Clinic doctors did not give him any other diagnosis than a chemical imbalance. He recalled being told that he would have to stay on the medicine for a long time.

I knew that Stelazine was a potent antipsychotic medication used primarily for schizophrenia [81], not a chemical imbalance in the brain, and I also knew that schizophrenia was most often diagnosed in young men from their late teens through their late twenties. Since Stelazine has many adverse side effects, another medicine, like Cogentin, often was started at the same time to minimize the substantial side effects of this antipsychotic medication.

On his first visit, Glen requested that I decrease the dose of his medications because he was feeling a lot better, that is, a lot less nervous, and he was too dopey in the morning before he went to work.

Since I did not know Glen and I didn't have any of his medical records, I did not feel it was appropriate to refill his prescription at half the dose and send him on his way. Therefore, I asked him to allow my office to obtain his records from the Mayo Clinic. In return, I would refill his prescription for several weeks at half the dose. After several weeks Glen was to return so we could go over his records from the Mayo Clinic together, and he could update me about how he was doing on the decreased medication dose. Glen agreed to my plan.

In the interim, my office received the psychiatric records from the Mayo Clinic where nothing was written about a suspected or confirmed diagnosis of schizophrenia. The only thing highlighted in the records was that he had a chemical imbalance in the brain. This became common psychiatry lingo starting in the 1970s for any psychiatric disorder. The identity of a chemical imbalance or whether one even exists has never been proven. The phrase is commonly used but remains a purely theoretical concept.

Glen returned about two weeks later and reported that he felt a lot better on the lower dose of medicine. In chatting with him, one never would suspect that Glen had a psychiatric problem. While talking, I asked questions about his daily life, his work, his medical history, and current events. All his answers seemed to be on point until I asked about current events. It just so happened that one of the space shuttle flights was in the current news. When I talked to Glen about the space shuttle flight, he got quite anxious. He asked me, "Do you know who the first man to land on the moon was?"

I replied, "Neil Armstrong."

Glen responded with excitement, "You're right." In rapid succession he asked, "How did they get to the moon?"

"On an Apollo spacecraft," I replied.

"Correct again." Glen exclaimed. "Now tell me, how do they figure out how to get the space ship to the moon?"

I answered that I knew onboard computers were used for navigation.

Glen responded, "And who do you think puts the information into the computers?"

I told Glen that I assumed the aerospace engineers entered programs into the computers.

To this comment he proclaimed, "No! I tell the engineers how to program the computers. I give them the mathematical information. I am the one the space engineers call to verify their computations. Now, what do you think about that?" I conveyed that I thought it was very interesting.

I could see that Glen was becoming agitated when he shouted, "I see you don't believe me. Here, I'll prove it to you." At this moment, Glen pulled a small spiral notebook from his back pocket, opened it, and gave it to me to evaluate.

The notebook had pictures drawn in pencil of the moon, the earth, lanes of orbit around the moon from the earth, and numerous mathematical calculations. There were separate sets of drawings and calculations for each Apollo space mission and each space shuttle mission up to the current space shuttle mission that was in the news. On the first page of the book I noticed three dates in large bold print under the title IMPORTANT: January 20, 1961, May 25, 1961, November 22, 1963. I asked Glen the significance of the dates.

With a bewildered stare, he emphatically informed me, "The first date was when John F. Kennedy was inaugurated as President of the United States. The second date was when John F. Kennedy said we would put a man on the moon by the end of the century. The third date was when President John F. Kennedy was assassinated in Dallas, Texas, by Lee Harvey Oswald." He then started to talk about all the calculations he had made, how often he received phone calls from the space engineers in Houston, Texas, regarding the current space shuttle mission, and how he checked all the calculations made by the spaceship computers with his own pencil before they were entered into the computers. Glen asserted that he had a direct communication line from the space shuttle to his house so he could check and monitor their calculations.

Obviously I quickly determined that my young patient was indeed delusional and most likely schizophrenic. It was interesting to me that the doctors at the Mayo Clinic had not mentioned Glen's space calculations. I thought that perhaps I had just hit the right trigger that day to get him started talking about his prowess in the space field.

Since Glen did not appear to me to be a danger to himself or to others and since he appeared to be able to live quite delightfully in his delusional state of being a space pioneer, I refilled his prescriptions for Stelazine and Cogentin for only three months that were to be dispensed one week at a time. I planned to see him every three months for reevaluations.

Over the next fifteen years Glen saw many more mental health caregivers. It seemed to me that he stayed with a single individual for no longer than a year or two. My office was able to obtain many records from these different mental health professionals; not one of them ever mentioned Glen's delusions of grandeur relating to the space program. None of these medical providers gave Glen a diagnosis other than a chemical abnormality in the brain. Most, however, freely added additional medications or changed his medications entirely in attempts to correct his chemical imbalance, whatever it was. [82, 83]

Glen continued to visit me in my office about once a year or so for various medical issues not related to his schizophrenia. As the years passed it became quite evident that Glen had a serious psychiatric disorder. He chain-smoked and had the yellow fingers to prove it. He started to wear foul smelling, dirty clothes, and his attention to personal hygiene essentially vanished. He grew withdrawn from society and was content to remain at home where he felt secure. Eventually, Glen developed the classic flat, expressionless face with wide-open eyes and a blank stare that often is seen in people with significant mental disease who use major psychiatric drugs.

It fascinated me that at each visit, Glen brought out the same little spiral notebook and repeated the same stories about how he was the mathematical wizard of the American space program. I was intrigued by Glen's perpetual delusions about space, so after a while I just sat back and listened to the same wonderful stories.

Wired

The Williston Basin is a large geologic formation that extends from the southern part of Saskatchewan in Canada almost five hundred miles south to the middle part of South Dakota and extends almost three hundred miles from east to west. Sidney, Montana, is situated directly over its center. Oil and gas reserves were first discovered in this formation near the turn of the twentieth century, and the first oil boom in the Williston Basin around Sidney occurred during the early 1950s.

The next oil boom in the Williston Basin started around 1975 during the few years of economic recovery following the Arab oil embargo in 1973. People from high unemployment areas all over the country ventured to eastern Montana and the western Dakotas searching for high-paying jobs in the oil fields. For about five years the economic activity in the Williston Basin was unprecedented. The influx of new people into the area strained municipal resources. The flow of money was prolific, and many people prospered. Unfortunately, a deep national economic recession started in early 1980 and essentially stopped all oil activities. Bank interest rates increased to twenty percent and more, and national unemployment rates eventually topped ten percent.

With an acute loss of jobs in the area, workers and their families left the oilfield communities by the thousands. One of the local bank presidents during this time told me that he hated to go to work on Monday mornings because during the weekends the outside deposit box at the bank, which was designated for loan payments, would be filled with keys for automobiles, homes, and all types of recreational vehicles that the oil field workers had purchased on credit. On their way out of town, the workers left their property with the banks because they had no money to pay the bills. The bank president told me that, in a very short period of time, the local banks not only lost considerable sums of money but also became the primary sellers of used automobiles, real estate, and used recreational vehicles of all sorts.

It was during this time that I became acquainted with Martha Ann and Raymond Stewart. This couple and their two children had come to Sidney from someplace in Texas searching for work. Raymond, who had experience working in the Texas oil fields, had little difficulty finding employment. Unfortunately, he was able to work for only a couple months before the recession hit our area.

After his shift ended on a Friday afternoon, Raymond was advised by his supervisor that his oil rig was shutting down, the company was closing down all its operations and leaving the Williston Basin, and all its employees were being laid off effective immediately. That night Raymond and Martha Ann discussed their situation, packed up their belongings, and planned to leave Sidney, Montana, and return to Texas the next morning.

Martha Ann was pregnant. For the short time her family had lived in Sidney, Martha Ann had not seen any local physician for prenatal care because the family had no money and no health insurance. All Martha Ann knew was the due date her last physician in Texas had given her was two weeks away.

Complicating her circumstances was the fact that Martha Ann had previously required surgery (cesarean section) to deliver her two children. Apparently, each operation was performed after she had gone into labor, and each time labor started exactly on her due date. Therefore, the pair naturally assumed that Martha Ann would start her labor in two weeks and figured they would have plenty of time to travel back to Texas before the baby had to be delivered.

The next morning was Saturday. While making breakfast for her children, Martha Ann felt some twinges in her abdomen. Soon thereafter the twinges became cramps. A short time later she noticed that the discomfort was recurring every few minutes and told Raymond they should wait before they left for Texas.

Raymond asked his wife if she was in labor. Martha Ann told him that she wasn't sure. However, she knew that she did not want to go into labor on a highway somewhere in the middle of nowhere in eastern Montana.

Raymond agreed, and the pair decided to wait for an hour to see what happened. As time passed, Martha Ann's cramps became more severe. She told her husband the pains were worse than she remembered and suggested that she go to the emergency room at the hospital to be checked.

I was the only physician in town delivering babies this particular weekend. The emergency room nurse reported that by the time Martha Ann arrived in our hospital she was definitely in a good labor pattern. She was having a substantial amount of pain with each contraction and confided to the nurse the pains were different and much worse compared to her other pregnancies. While monitoring the woman's labor, the nurse checked the fetal heart tones and performed a pelvic examination. She reported to me that Martha Ann's labor was of good quality with a regular pattern, the baby's heart tones were normal and did not show a pattern of fetal distress, and the patient's cervix was starting to dilate. After this conversation, I asked the nurse to transfer Martha Ann to the obstetric area where I would meet her as soon as possible.

When I met the parents-to-be in her room in the obstetrics wing of the hospital, Raymond had their two children with him. The nurse who accompanied me into the room escorted the children to our hospital playroom after the parents gave her their permission.

After introducing myself to the couple and reading the information on my new patient's chart, I took a brief history from Martha Ann about her previous pregnancies. I learned that her first operation occurred after the baby had signs of distress. The second operation resulted from her being unable to deliver the baby naturally. Martha Ann said her last doctor told her that she would need an operation with all of her future babies. My patient told me she did not take any medicines except vitamins, she did not drink alcohol, and she did not use tobacco products.

I noticed my patient appeared to be having considerable discomfort with each of her contractions. Martha Ann mentioned to me, as she had done with the nurse in the emergency room, that her pains were much worse than those in her previous pregnancies. My findings on physical examination matched those of the emergency room nurse. I informed the couple that indeed Martha Ann was in labor and that I should perform an operation to deliver the baby. I informed the pair that I would notify the surgical team promptly, and we should be able to have the operation completed within the next couple of hours.

I told Martha Ann that because of the short time before she delivered I would not be giving her any medication for pain. Furthermore, I informed her that our anesthetist on duty did not administer regional anesthesia. Consequently, she would have to be put to sleep for the operation, and I gave her the general description of how the procedure would be performed. Martha Ann responded that she had received general anesthesia with her two previous operations and was not worried.

I walked to the nurse's station and telephoned the anesthetist and the surgical team members. They informed me that I should be able to operate within half an hour, so I returned to my patient's room and relayed my conversations to the couple. I then went to the hospital's medical records department to complete some records while I waited for the surgical team to prepare Martha Ann for surgery.

When Martha Ann was in the operating room and being readied for surgery, I inspected the newborn resuscitation equipment and the incubator with the nursery nurse who had been called in for the surgery. All the emergency equipment was functioning satisfactorily. I routinely checked the equipment before every delivery and every C-section.

While I scrubbed my hands before surgery, the surgical assistants cleaned Martha Ann's swollen abdomen and placed sterile drapes around her. After donning my sterile surgical gown and gloves, I asked each person in the operating room if they were ready to go. I then leaned over and asked Martha Ann if she was ready to have a baby. She replied, "I'm ready if you are Doctor."

The anesthetist asked me to give her a few moments to get our patient ready and said she would tell me when I could start. As usual, I told her that we couldn't do anything until she was ready. I asked her to just let us know when we could begin the operation.

When the anesthetist asked me to proceed gently, I made a skin incision with a scalpel beside the old vertical incision which barely opened the skin from near the belly button toward pubic bone. The next cut with the scalpel went deeper into the fatty tissue just beneath the skin. Immediately I felt and heard a thud under the scalpel blade. I thought to myself, "What the heck?" I asked the surgical assistant if she heard the noise, but she denied hearing anything.

My next motion with the scalpel produced a similar noise with a similar obstruction to my scalpel's progress. I looked closer at the fatty tissue and noticed that the entire incision had been closed previously with wire. This time I said out loud, "What the heck?" I showed the wire to the surgical technician who looked puzzled and noted that she had never seen wire in the fat tissue like that before.

I asked the surgical technician if she happened to have any wire cutters on her surgical instrument table. She replied, "Dr. A, you're kidding me, aren't you? This is a C-section." Looking at her, I said, "Well, I need to cut the wire somehow. Do you have any heavy bandage scissors?" The surgical assistant asked me to wait two seconds. She then reached under a nearby set of drapes and pulled out a pair of heavy bandage scissors. She said, "I won't let you ruin my good new bandage scissors. However, you can use this pair the orthopedic surgeon ruined cutting bones." She handed me a pair of heavy-duty scissors.

The wire in the fatty tissue was of a small enough gauge that the heavy scissors cut through the sutures easily. Opening the fatty tissue layer entirely exposed the next layer of fibrous tissue (the fascia), which had been put together at the previous surgery with heavy wire staples. I said out loud, "What kind of obstetrician would put his patient together with staples?"

It was obvious to me that the heavy scissors were not going to cut through the numerous heavy metal staples. Since time was of the essence in getting out the baby, I elected to bypass the metal staples on one side to open up the patient's abdomen.

After performing this maneuver, I was able to enter my patient's abdomen without any more difficulty. Upon opening the abdomen and exposing the pregnant uterus, the surgical technician and I both saw a uterus that had been stapled shut during her last operation. Neither the surgical technician nor I had ever seen such a wound closure. Fortunately for me, the surgical technician, after witnessing the size of the metal sutures in the fascia, had the operating room supervisor procure a large staple-removing instrument. When she put this tool in front of me, I just looked at her with joy. She said, "Here, doctor, maybe this will help."

While I was removing the staples in the pregnant uterus, I mentioned to the surgical team that I thought I understood why my patient was having more labor pain than usual.

The staple-removing instrument worked well. After the staple sutures were removed, I was able to open my patient's uterus, extract a healthy female infant without difficulty, and hand a screaming baby to the nursery nurse waiting nearby. The surgical supervisor informed me that, despite all the difficulties, I was still able to deliver the baby within four minutes. I thanked her for her good report, but my brain felt as if it had taken hours.

In the process of completing the operation, the surgical technician and I removed every fragment of wire and every wire staple we could find and placed the pieces into a specimen container. I asked the surgical supervisor to label the container for my patient because I wanted to show her why I thought she had such severe pain.

The remainder of the operation was not remarkable, thank goodness. The anesthetist had administered a marvelous general anesthesia, and Martha Ann awakened just a few moments after I completed closing her skin wound and while I was applying a bandage. She asked how her baby was. I told Martha Ann that she was fine, her baby was fine, and the operation went without a hitch. The last part certainly was a stretch of the truth. I had the nursery nurse bring the newborn infant next to the new mom's face so they could see each other.

Afterward when I went out to tell Raymond that all was well, he thanked me, but he appeared to be concerned about something, so I asked what was bothering him. Raymond explained that he and his two kids did not have a place to stay, he did not have any money to rent a motel room, and he wanted to know how long Martha Ann would be in the hospital. That's when he revealed they had no money and no health insurance since he lost his job.

I told Raymond to enjoy the moment. I would see what I could do to make some arrangements for him and his children.

I then talked to the hospital's charge nurse about the Stewart family's dilemma. Dismissing the problem, the nurse explained that there were empty beds on the obstetrics wing that could be used as a family room for a short time. Meals from the cafeteria could be added to Martha Ann's hospital bill, which probably wouldn't be paid anyway because of the family's financial situation. Finally, the children had toys to keep them occupied in the playroom. The nurse figured the family could stay at the hospital for a week easily, if needed.

The next day I asked Martha Ann who had performed her last operation. She replied that an older general surgeon in a small town in Texas did it. I suggested, but could not confirm, that her increased pain might have been caused by her tissues trying to stretch around, or being torn by, the metal staples we found during surgery.

Knowing that the Stewart family would be traveling to Texas soon after the new mom and baby were discharged from the hospital, I kept the family in the hospital for about a week. During that time, I raided the hospital's nursery and my office for samples of baby formula. Luckily, the Mead Johnson sales representative, who sold the infant formula Enfamil, came by my office. After I presented Martha Ann's story to him, he generously left several cases of infant formula for the new baby.

Martha Ann's convalescence was unremarkable. I discharged her and her baby the next Saturday and wished the family well in their journey. I gave her the metal staples and the wires as souvenirs from her experience in Sidney, Montana.

On Monday morning I asked my office employees not to send the Raymond family a bill because I figured they would not know where to send it, I would not be paid anyhow, and the parents had enough to worry about.

The Long Goodbye

My family and I had been in Sidney, Montana, for just a short time when one of my neighbors invited me to attend one of the weekly cattle sales at the local auction yard. He and I arrived at the sales yard about six o'clock in the morning so my neighbor could introduce me to some of his friends and neighbors living in and around Sidney. On this day, there was to be a larger than usual cattle sale, and a throng of people, both buyers and sellers, had congregated in the bleachers surrounding the sales arena.

One of the notable people that I met this day was Jack Grearson, a local man who owned a farm and ranch operation a short distance from town. My first impression of Jack was that he was a soft-spoken and mild-mannered fellow who was quite intelligent and articulate. I guessed that Jack was perhaps in his late thirties or early forties. I had the opportunity to speak with Jack for only a short time before my neighbor introduced me to more people, and Jack had some work to do before he sold his cattle.

While eating breakfast before the cattle auction and while driving home after the sale, my neighbor and I discussed many topics. In particular, he talked about Jack Grearson favorably. He thought that Jack had a mind like a steel trap and, despite barely getting through high school, he was smart. He was not book smart, but he could repair or rebuild any of his farm machinery without a manual. "Jack," my neighbor said, "may not be able to read a book very well, but he can read animals with the best of them." My neighbor mentioned that, in his view, Jack was particularly good at caring for horses and cattle.

Jack was not a social animal according to my neighbor, but he did okay in groups. Jack usually didn't say much, yet when he did, people listened because they knew he meant what he said. My neighbor also noted, "I learned not to underestimate Jack's ability to observe things. He can read people just as good as he reads his animals."

Later in our conversations my neighbor again talked about Jack. He said Jack had an incredible memory and could recall the face and name of just about anyone he had ever met. He could remember the price that cattle sold for years before. He could remember specific things related to his farm, such as the precipitation totals from years past, the amount of fertilizer he had used per acre on each field on his farm, his farm yields of grain for many years past, and so on.

I had the opportunity to talk with Jack on several occasions over the next ten years, but not in a professional capacity. Besides his many attributes, Jack was extremely healthy. During these visits I found that my neighbor's initial comments about Jack were all true. His brain was photographic and contained an amazing amount of information that he was able to access with little difficulty. Even though Jack did not read very much, whatever he did read, his brain retained quickly for future reference. Whatever he heard or observed, his brain stored it for a later use. Likewise, whatever he touched, smelled, or felt emotionally, I was convinced that Jack's brain could store this information and retrieve it just as easily.

One day, one of Jack's sons asked if I would mind talking to his dad because he thought something was wrong. The son admitted that he couldn't put his finger on exactly what was wrong, but it seemed to him that Jack's memory was failing, and his dad was only fifty years old. I asked the son to have Jack visit me in my clinic. I suggested to him that perhaps I would be able to do some testing informally to determine if Jack was having some issues with his memory. The son agreed to bring his father into my clinic the next week.

When I saw Jack in my clinic, we just talked as we had done before, yet I noticed right away that he was having a little difficulty retrieving common, everyday information. The changes in his mental function, however, appeared to be minimal after we chatted for perhaps an hour. Afterward I thought Jack might have had a small stroke or that he was showing the early stages of a dementia. I knew that only time would tell what was really happening.

I presented my observations and thoughts to the son and asked him to keep good notes of his father's behavior and to follow-up with me or another physician every three months. He promised to keep a diary.

Jack's wife and son visited with me again about four years later. They informed me that Jack had been diagnosed with Alzheimer's disease[84, 85] two years earlier and had been started on a prescription medication that was going to stop the progress of his disease and make things better. They asked if I would refill Jack's prescription for his Alzheimer's medication.

I asked the pair if they had noticed any improvement in Jack's thought processes or behavior since he started taking the medicine. They told me that they had not. In fact, Jack seemed to be getting worse. However, Jack's doctor, who was a neurologist, encouraged them to give the medicine some time to work. I asked them, "How long is some time? It's been two years." They did not know the answer. The neurologist reassured them with his optimism and just kept writing the prescriptions, which, by the way, cost them about $250 per month.

From my experience and the medical literature and contrary to the glowing results portrayed in advertisements on television and other media, I told Jack's wife and son that the medicines for Alzheimer's disease did not produce any noticeable clinical improvement in the dementia nor in the natural progression of the disease process.[86] I told them bluntly that if the medicine was not working after two years, it wasn't going to work. I gave them some references they could obtain from a computer, the public library, or the local pharmacist to verify my comments.

The wife became upset with me when I told her that her husband realistically was not going to improve. Crying, she told me that taking care of him the last couple years had been a nightmare. Every morning it seemed that she had lost another piece of her Jack during the night. She related to me that her husband was no longer mild-mannered, but got upset with minimal provocation. She explained that some days she had to remind her husband how to use a knife and a fork. Furthermore, the wife added that Jack was having other problems. She revealed to me he slept poorly, had difficulty eating, felt tired all the time, and complained of a lot of muscle cramps in his legs.

I attributed these symptoms to possible adverse side effects of his medications and told her so.

The son interjected that his father no longer could remember how to run the farm equipment or how to put seed in the grain drills. On top of this, the son related how his father would get mad at him for no apparent reason and, at times, was angry enough to try to hit him.

Again I sympathized with the pair but repeated that the medicine was not working and that it was not going to work. Jack's dementia, if it were Alzheimer's disease, would continue unchecked by any medication, and eventually he would require round-the-clock care. I suggested that they discuss Jack's situation with the people at our local nursing home because I knew it had a dementia ward and employees specially trained to care for clients with end-stage dementia.

After these comments, both the wife and the son became irate with me and accused me of not caring. I tried to explain to the pair that I was just trying to give them a realistic view of what they could and should expect from Jack's disease in the future. After this visit, I had no further contact with Jack or his family.

About two years later, I received a letter from Jack's wife. In the letter she wrote that she had read that Alzheimer's disease was called the long goodbye, and now she understood why. She went on to recall how she and her family had struggled with Jack's disease since I had talked with them several years before. She apologized for not believing me then because, as she said, "We weren't ready to believe it." She wanted to believe the medicines were going to cure her husband. She explained in her letter that the family had finally decided to place Jack into a nursing home the previous week because they could no longer care for him at home.

She finished her note by writing, “Seven years dealing with Jack’s Alzheimer's on a daily basis was indeed a very long goodbye.” She signed her note, “Sincerely and gratefully yours, Mrs. Jack Grearson.”

EPILOGUE

"A good day is one in which you give something to someone for which they can never repay you."

John Wooden

Epilogue

The advancement of medical knowledge through the ages has been a long, often tedious, yet unwavering, process. Just like early physicians who we now believe had misguided ideas and questionable treatments, modern medicine might well be the victim of the same opinions by future generations. We cannot deny, however, that health care around the world at the turn of the twenty-first century is better than ever before. Mostly because of the improvements in sanitation and childhood survival, the median life expectancy at birth in America has improved from about thirty-eight years in 1800 to about seventy-nine years two hundred years later. Furthermore, if a child lived to the age of ten years in 1800, the life expectancy increased to about sixty years. [87] I wonder if a physician in colonial Virginia in the 1700s could have dreamed of such improvement? I also wonder if there is an endpoint to this medical progress. Does the human body have an age after which it cannot survive?

Perhaps we will become like the buggy in Oliver Wendell Holmes' poem, "The Deacon's Masterpiece" or "The Wonderful One-Hoss Shay." The deacon built a two-person carriage with each part as strong as the next so it would not break down. The carriage lasted one hundred years to the day before it disintegrated into a pile of dust. [88]

Through the centuries many have sought the source of immortality, a Fountain of Youth, and failed. Will science in the future help us find such a place, or will we come to the realization, like many have before us, that there is no Fountain of Youth?

Now that our genetic code has been cracked and the human genome deciphered, what knowledge and tools await future physicians to attack known and unknown diseases with more disease-specific treatments? [89, 90]

For now, as in the past, physicians and scientists will continue to face many more new and different challenges. There will be new and different diseases like AIDS and SARS (Severe Acute Respiratory Syndrome). Doctors and scientists will face challenges from old germs with new faces and new microbes that have not yet been discovered. The lifelong treatment of the physical and mental injuries resulting from wars will continue to challenge us. The perpetual struggles with the many medical and social problems confronting our increasingly aging population, such as dementia, heart disease, cancer, and overall body wasting, will continue to accelerate.[91]

In the years ahead, everyone will witness and experience side effects in one form or another. With the changes coming to our scientific understanding of diseases and to medical care, it is inevitable that side effects will occur; as in the past, some will be beneficial, some harmful, and some catastrophic.

Winston Churchill wrote, "The greatest refinements of science are linked with the cruelties of the stone age." Was he right?

Throughout this inexorable chaotic process of scientific and medical advancement with all its side effects, both good and bad, there will continue to be at least one constant. There will always be the patients who will look to their physician for help in relieving their suffering; there will continue to be physicians who treat sick and injured people with the hopes and expectations that they can and will make their patients better.

Bibliography

Prologue

1. Every Man His Own Doctor: OR, The Poor Planter's Physician, 1734, Dr. John Tenant, original pamphlet printed by Benjamin Frankin, Philadelphia, 1734, Facsimile reprint by Colonial Williamsburg Foundation Press, 2011
2. Opium Poppy: History
3. Cinchona - Wikipedia
4. St. John's Wort,www.herballegacy.com/Nelson_History
5. History of St. John's Wort, google search
6. Urban Herbs: Foxglove
7. Side effect - Wikipedia

Old Blue Eyes

8. Viagra: A Chronology
9. The Road to Sildenafil – A history of artificial erections
10. History of Viagra | Sildenafil aka Viagra
11. Complications and risks of Viagra | SteadyHealth.com
12. Viagra Side Effects | Drugs.com

One Hairy Adventure

13. Minoxidil - oral (Loniten) side effects, medical uses, and drug interactions.
14. Loniten Official FDA information, side effects and uses.
15. The History of Rogaine | eHow.com
16. The unusual history of Minoxidil
17. Minoxidil Mini-Series: Part 2 – From Blood Pressure to Baldness
18. Minoxidil - Wikipedia
19. History of The Upjohn Company

More Than Meets The Eye

20. Timolol - Wikipedia
21. Timolol Ophthalmic: MedlinePlus Drug Information
22. Timeless Timolol?
23. Should beta blockers be abandoned as initial monotherapy in chronic open angle glaucoma?

Bad Medicine

24. Selacryn (Drug) - Detailed Information
25. Selacryn legal admission

Jump Start

26. Amiodarone - Google Search
27. Amiodarone Information from Drugs.com
28. Cortisone - Wikipedia
29. Cortisone Top : Uses, Side Effects, Interactions, Pictures, Warnings & Dosing - WebMD

Too Many Pills

30. Plavix (clopidogrel) Information from Drugs.com
31. Clopidogrel - Wikipedia
32. Statin Therapy and the Elderly
33. http:// Statins for women, elderly
34. Welcome to the UCSD Statin Effects Study
35. Beta blocker - Wikipedia
36. The Relationship of Dietary Fat and Cholesterol to Mortality in 10 Years: The Honolulu Heart Program

Elephants and Dragons

37. Delirium tremens: MedlinePlus Medical Encyclopedia
38. Delirium tremens - Wikipedia
39. Delirium tremens - PubMed

Just Kill Me Now

40. Apomorphine: MedlinePlus Drug Information
41. Apomorphine - Wikipedia,

Juan Juice

42. Effects of LSD - What Are the Effects of LSD?
43. Lysergic acid diethylamide (LSD) - Wikipedia

It's All Your Fault

44. Timeline of AIDS - Wikipedia
45. History of HIV & AIDS in the United States of America
46. HIV/AIDS - Wikipedia
47. HIV in the United States | Fact sheets
48. Cost Of Treatment Still A Challenge For HIV Patients In U.S.

49. AIDS patients will spend $600K for care - Health - AIDS | NBC News
50. Aging with AIDS: Living longer, living with loss - Health - AIDS | NBC News

A Bit of Luck

51. A history of neonatal group B streptococcus w... [J Pediatric Nursing. 2004
52. Group B streptococcal infection - Wikipedia,
53. Group B streptococcal septicemia of the newborn: MedlinePlus
54. Prenatal screening for group B streptococcal infection: gaps in the evidence
55. Group B Strep in pregnancy review

Old Dog, New Trick

56. Lexicomp Newsletter-aspirin
57. History of aspirin - Wikipedia,
58. History of Aspirin

A False Test

59. Reviving the Acid Phosphatase Test for Prostate Cancer-Cancer Network
60. Prostate-specific antigen, Wikipedia
61. Halting PSA testing the right thing to do, bioethicist says
62. PSA Tests | Wellness Letter
63. Prostatic cancer: Further Investigation of Hormonal Relationships Incidence and Mortality, Prostate Cancer Trends, 1973-1995

Help Me Breathe

64. Bubbles, Babies and Biology: The Story of Surfactant
65. Pulmonary surfactant - Wikipedia
66. Surfactant Deficiency | Child Foundation
67. Mary Ellen Avery, Premature Babies' Savior, Dies at 84 - NYTimes.com
68. Infant Mortality Rates, 1950–2005 —
69. Infant Mortality US 19352007.doc

Three Women

70. DCIS - Ductal Carcinoma In Situ

71. The Confusion Over DCIS: What to Do About 'Stage Zero' Breast Cancer?
72. Compass: Ductal Carcinoma In Situ
73. Breast Cancer Topic: Percentage of False-Positive Mammograms
74. Prone to Error - Earliest Steps to Find Cancer - NYTimes.com
75. Cancer of the Breast - SEER Stat Fact Sheets
76. Natural History of Breast Cancer
77. Natural history of breast cancers detected in t... [Lancet Oncology. 2011]
78. The natural history of breast cancer, ncbi.nlm.nih.gov/pubmed/10572545

Sam

79. Parkinson's disease - MayoClinic.com
80. Parkinson's disease - Wikipedia

Space Wizard

81. Schizophrenia - wikipedia
83. The Illusions of Psychiatry by Marcia Angell | The New York Review of Books
82. The Epidemic of Mental Illness: Why? by Marcia Angell | The New York Review of Books

The Long Goodbye

84. Alzheimer's disease - Wikipedia
85. Alzheimer's disease - PubMed Health
86. Alzheimer's Disease Medications Fact Sheet | National Institute on Aging Do Medications for the Treatment of Alzheimer's Disease Work?

Epilogue

87. Life expectancy in the 1800s not as bad as reported
88. The Deacon's Masterpiece - Wikisource
89. Computing the Genome
90. Genetic code - Wikipedia
91. Make More Room: Nursing Home Population Set To Explode.

*** All resources can be found with Google or another electronic search engine

Made in United States
North Haven, CT
09 March 2026

89674124R00136